The Rhythms of W D0446118

◎ ◎ ◎

Praise for Elizabeth Davis's work

"A gold mine! It contains heart and soul and information…never encountered before in any form. A potent and appreciative chronicle of what it means to be a woman at home in her body…the more women (and men, for that matter) who read this, the more quickly our world will be healed."

— *Isabella*

"When a book on sex comes along that you think your own doctor should read, you may want to order up extra copies and pass them around at your next appointment! Enormously refreshing."

— *Libido*

"An appealing mixture of medically sound fact, thorough female intuition, underhanded humor and sensitivity…could surprise and educate even the most sexually seasoned people."

— *Moving Words/Moving Books*

"Elizabeth Davis writes vividly, succinctly, and joyously. [She] reveals a shrewd and compassionate sensitivity to women's needs…"

— Sheila Kitzinger
Author of *The Experience of Childbirth,*
The Complete Book of Pregnancy and Birth,
and *The Place of Birth*

"Elizabeth…the wisdom of your work is as old as time."

— Christiane Northrup, MD
Author of *Women's Bodies, Women's Wisdom*

DEDICATION

*I dedicate this book to my beloved daughter, Celeste,
and to all women determined to love their bodies
and own their power, no matter the cost.
Particularly to those in parts of the world where oppression
makes this very difficult, I pay tribute to your acts
of vision and courage.*

◎   ◎   ◎

About the Author

ELIZABETH DAVIS has been a midwife and women's
health-care provider since 1977. She is co-director of
the National Midwifery Institute, Inc. and instructor of
Heart and Hands Midwifery Intensive courses. She is
the author of many successful books, including *Orgasmic
Birth: Your Guide to a Safe, Satisfying and Pleasurable Birth
Experience; The Women's Wheel of Life;* and *Heart and
Hands: A Midwife's Guide to Pregnancy and Birth,* now in
its 5th edition. She lectures internationally to midwives,
nurses, gynecologists, and obstetricians on subjects related to women's health, psychology, and reproductive
issues. She lives in Sebastopol, CA, and is the mother of
three children, grandmother of one.

Ordering

Trade bookstores in the U.S. and Canada please contact
Publishers Group West
1700 Fourth Street, Berkeley CA 94710
Phone: (800) 788-3123   Fax: (800) 351-5073

For bulk orders please contact
Special Sales
Hunter House Inc., PO Box 2914, Alameda CA 94501-0914
Phone: (510) 899-5041   Fax: (510) 865-4295
E-mail: sales@hunterhouse.com

Individuals can order our books by calling **(800) 266-5592**
or from our website at **www.hunterhouse.com**

The
Rhythms *of*
Women's Desire

How Female Sexuality Unfolds
at Every Stage of Life

Elizabeth Davis

With a Foreword by Germaine Greer

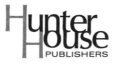

Hunter House
PUBLISHERS

Copyright © 2013 by Elizabeth Davis

Hunter House Inc., Publishers
PO Box 2914
Alameda CA 94501-0914

Library of Congress Cataloging-in-Publication Data

Davis, Elizabeth, 1950-
[Women's sexual passages]
The rhythms of women's desire : how female sexuality unfolds at every stage of life / Elizabeth Davis ; with a foreword by Germaine Greer. — Third Edition.
pages cm
Revision of the author's Women's sexual passages.
Includes bibliographical references and index.
ISBN 978-0-89793-650-7 (pbk.) — ISBN 978-0-89793-651-4 (ebk.)
1. Women — Sexual behavior. 2. Women — Physiology. 3. Hormones, Sex — Physiological effect. 4. Women — Health and hygiene. I. Title.
HQ29.D294 2013
306.7082 — dc23   2012041750

Project Credits
Cover Design: Peri Poloni-Gabriel
Book Production: John McKercher
Copy Editor: Susan Lyn McCombs
Indexer: Candace Hyatt
Managing Editor: Alexandra Mummery
Acquisitions Coordinator: Susan Lyn McCombs
Editorial Intern: Tu-Anh Dang-Tran
Special Sales Manager: Judy Hardin
Publicity Coordinator: Martha Scarpati
Rights Coordinator: Candace Groskreutz
Publisher's Assistant: Bronwyn Emery
Customer Service Manager: Christina Sverdrup
Order Fulfillment: Washul Lakdhon
Administrator: Theresa Nelson
Computer Support: Peter Eichelberger
Publisher: Kiran S. Rana

Printed and bound by Bang Printing, Brainerd, Minnesota
Manufactured in the United States of America

9 8 7 6 5 4 3 2 1   Third Edition   13 14 15 16 17

Contents

Foreword

In the postwar years of the twentieth century, the power of the female stereotype was exponentially extended and intensified by mass marketing until brassieres and high heels, nail polish and lipstick were to be found in every hovel on the globe. As the stereotype's grip tightened, resistance was born. It gathered, swelled, burst through underground channels and up into the consciousness of real women outraged and baffled by the conflicting demands made upon them. The struggle to vomit up the internalized guilt and the ingrained certainties of defect and inadequacy is not over, because male fantasy is still the deciding factor in our buying and selling. The breast-popping stereotype still dangles her four-foot legs off the car hood. The icon of the dazzling supermenial whose hands never say housework, who is always accessible to the penis and climaxes whenever her partner does (and is never without a desirous partner), and never falters on the rope bridge over the chasm of parenting, is still displayed in all our houses. But her stranglehold on female variety is gradually being loosened. Gay women have defied her way up front. Heterosexual women too, have steadily, quietly rewritten the agenda to include singleness, aging, aggression, wit, and sorrow. Character has been inscribed upon the smooth, featureless skin of the female stereotype as women have demanded the right to grow up and turn into people.

The great tension at the heart of feminism has always been the pull to demand entry to the male world, and claim an equal share of male characteristics, against the pressure for the right to be different but not inferior. Some feminists argued for the industrialization of motherhood and the right to carry arms in imperialist wars and to direct the bone-crushing operations of multinationals. Others wondered what real femaleness might be like, as distinct from prescribed femininity. They moved into the inscape of the gendered body, deconstructing biological femaleness not as a defect, not as a distortion of a male norm by the specific imperatives of childbearing, but as a complex and variable norm in itself. They took to heart the biological lesson that it is not the female but the male that is the product of a defective gene.

A gifted and persistent group of women professionals set themselves the task of observing first hand how female humans really do behave. They discovered that all kinds of received ideas about female anatomy were simply wrong, that all kinds of variations were contained within a normality far more capacious than anyone had realized before. Gradually the conviction that femaleness is a permanent disease began to lose its hold. Fathers rose from attending birthing women with a new respect for their resilience and power. Women turned away from the hospital and the clinic, looking for ways to take responsibility for their own wellbeing. Feminist observers put together a picture of a hitherto unknown creature, the well woman.

We still have a long way to go; the medical establishment still labors under the delusion that femaleness is a condition that demands treatment, that women's fertility is the cause of overpopulation, that machines are better at birthing than women, that wombs are something that should be extirpated, and that the menstrual cycle involves periodic insanity.

Elizabeth Davis has given women the kind of patient, loving, and respectful attention that is usually reserved for rhinos and mountain gorillas. Here is a practitioner who does not prescribe but describes, in terms that are both empowering and fascinating, the extraordinary inventiveness and variety of the human female in all her moods and phases.

— Germaine Greer

Author's Note

This book springs from a desire to help women understand and enjoy their sexuality, no matter what their age or situation. We now recognize that life is more than a continuum of experience; instead, it is comprised of stages distinct from one another and often age-linked. This overview of women's sexuality not only explores changes by decade but also highlights the physiological turning points of menarche, childbirth, and menopause. These climactic events have been called Blood Mysteries, as the change they render in our lives is both rapid and striking. The scope of transformation that occurs with each of these events and the similarities between them has long fascinated me and motivated my research, and I'm pleased to have an opportunity to present my findings.

This is also a book about honoring desire and sexual pleasure. Too often, stress and overwork push pleasure away, or if negative conditioning is a factor, guilt may interfere. But pleasure is important: Particularly in challenging times, we cannot find balance without it. In order to really know pleasure, we must continually re-explore what works for us, redefining our personal blend of relaxation, stimulation, and release. Note that the hormonal changes of the Blood Mysteries prompt dramatic shifts in this pleasure equation. The better we know our bodies and ourselves, the greater our chance of discovering the right mix as our lives unfold.

For most women, the greatest pleasure of all comes from intimacy in deep connection to another. Connection is the focal point of women's desire. The more we learn about neurobiology, the more we recognize this female predilection as natural and body-based. Not only in love but also in life, women want the big picture and are endlessly fascinated by how things connect and interrelate. For example, consider our usual approach to problem solving: We seek to incorporate as many factors as possible, deliberately soliciting conflicting viewpoints in order to get to the heart of the matter and distill core truth. This is what author Helen Fisher has termed "web thinking."[1]

This tendency may be linked to brain evolution. In primordial times, women's ability to pay attention to many things simultaneously and still stay alert was essential to rearing young in somewhat threatening circumstances. With a baby on her hip, other children clamoring for her attention, food preparation under way, and some wild beast scuffling just outside the door, a woman had to be expert at diffusing her attention as she multitasked for survival. Men, on the other hand, had to stay highly focused, single-minded in hunting or defending self and kin. Women's aptitude for contextual, holistic thinking has led, over time, to high expectations of their sexual partners. In their desire for complex communication, layer upon layer, no wonder it is challenging for women today to find the depth of intimacy they long for.

Deep intimacy is understandably elusive in a society that defines sexual pleasure in terms of technique and role-playing. Most of us have had our fill of that. Nevertheless, intimacy will elude us unless we are fully intimate with ourselves. It's interesting how persistently we seek to be close to others, and yet often avoid our own fears or limitations in this regard. Yet if we long for deep intimacy and its fruits of pleasure, we must undertake the quest for self-knowledge and self-love.

How did I come to write this book? I have been a midwife, well-woman care provider, and health educator for more than thirty years, with ample opportunity to hear women's sexual stories and treat their concerns. Many of my observations and much of my data have been gleaned from my work with childbearing women: As a midwife, I provide not only physical care but also a large measure of education and counseling. As a mother of three, I know firsthand that pregnancy, birth, and postpartum are vulnerable times for a woman, as rapid change and adjustment may lead to sexual estrangement.

The need for this book became increasingly clear as I opened my practice to women of all ages, from those not yet sexually active to those well beyond menopause. Thus I have been privy to the confidences and confessions of hundreds of women, sharing not only current concerns but also early, formative experiences. Many of my clients have had technical questions about their bodies; for example, women getting off the Pill often wonder about how this might affect their sex drive, and then become concerned about changes in vaginal secretion during the monthly cycle that are entirely normal. Similarly, perimenopausal women ask about hot flashes, vaginal dryness, and dramatically fluctuating levels of desire. I find these questions to be surprisingly basic, and as I continue to hear them repeatedly, I am alarmed to think how little even the most sophisticated women know about their bodies, their hormones, and their sexual makeup.

Sometimes I am faced with questions that are much more complex, involving loss of desire under circumstances of chronic stress, grief, history of abuse, or relationship upheavals. It is obvious that the bits and pieces of information most women have regarding their sexuality are not sufficient to meet their needs. So, here is my attempt to provide an overview of sexual desire and response, and a context both feminine and feminist, that links hormonal influences, the Blood Mysteries, and changes by stage of life.

My clients have enlightened me and have also helped me better understand myself. I, too, have increasingly learned to trust my instincts, my body-borne wisdom. This has led me to a greater appreciation and trust of women in general, and to a firm belief in our capacity for self-care. Whatever problem a woman may have, I believe she herself holds the keys to its solution. It's my task to help her find relevant information and adequate support for her healing process. For example, I've discovered that women in labor usually know better than I how to advance progress, whether through increased privacy, rest, or deep reassurance. Beyond monitoring the physical wellbeing of mother and child, my primary role is to enable the laboring woman to trust her instincts and ask for what she needs. The same is true in assisting nonpregnant women who are considering elective surgical procedures, or debating whether to use allopathic medicine or alternative therapies. I know women's strength and resourcefulness—I've witnessed it time and again.

And I decry the fact that women have been so shortchanged, handicapped by cultural mores that reduce their value to physical attractiveness. What a loss for all of us, that women's remarkable and exquisite complexity has been belittled and diminished by society. Yet I don't consider it premature to say that this mind-set is in decline. Although the change is nearly imperceptible in some parts of the world, the paradigm of women as the second sex is waning. Why now?

Helen Fisher, author of *The First Sex*, holds this vision of our future:

> *As women continue to pour into the paid workforce in cultures around the world, they will apply their natural aptitudes in many sectors of society and dramatically influence twenty-first century business, sex, and family life. In some important parts of the economy, they will even predominate, becoming the first sex. Why? Because current trends in business, communications, education, law, medicine, government and the nonprofit sector, known as civil society, all suggest that tomorrow's world will need the female mind.*[2]

Internet technology has utterly transformed our world. Communication has not only accelerated but has also completely outgrown linear parameters. The Web *is* a web! And the business that organizes around its use must employ contextual thinking, at which women so readily excel. Thus, it is no exaggeration to say that the future depends on women's inborn abilities to incorporate diversity, take the long view, survive ambiguity, and choose love.

The personal accounts in *The Rhythms of Women's Desire* paraphrase comments made by my clients over the years, plus recent interview responses solicited through my women's health practice. Words cannot express the gratitude I feel toward all who have contributed to this project.

My deepest wish is that this book be useful, that it inspire women to set aside self-doubt and teach their partners, and their children, a true view of women's nature where the sexual aspect is no longer isolated and exploited but rather, integrated and free. Let us build trust by sharing knowledge—as women have always done.

Important Note

The material in this book is intended to provide a review of information regarding women's sexuality and sexual health. Every effort has been made to provide accurate and dependable information. The contents of this book have been compiled through professional research and in consultation with medical and mental-health professionals. However, health-care professionals have differing opinions, and advances in medical and scientific research are made very quickly, so some of the information may become outdated.

Therefore, the publisher, authors, and editors, as well as the professionals quoted in the book, cannot be held responsible for any error, omission, or dated material. The authors and publisher assume no responsibility for any outcome of applying the information in this book in a program of self-care or under the care of a licensed practitioner. If you have questions concerning the information described in this book, consult a qualified health-care professional.

CHAPTER 1

Women, Sex, *and* Culture

If you have ever been puzzled by your sexual mood swings, your whims, fantasies, and aversions, this book is for you! Women in civilized society have increasingly lost touch with their natural rhythms of desire, particularly in cultures dominated by male values and attitudes. Virtually our only popular reference to female sexual rhythms is a negative one, that of the undesirability of menstruating women. We will explore this taboo in depth, along with others regarding pregnancy, menopause, and sex in later years. But first, we must define the cultural milieu that conditions our view of women's bodies and sexuality in such negative and condescending ways.

Experts on the evolution of patriarchy tell us the trouble began with the advent of an agrarian lifestyle. When we gave up our hunter-gatherer existence in favor of tending and cultivating land, ownership became an issue—particularly for men, who sought to transfer property to their male offspring. This led to claiming ownership of the mothers of their children.

Organized religion has not helped women's struggle for equality. In the time of the Spanish Inquisition (1400 to 1600 AD), their status in society had greatly deteriorated. Now considered to be unclean, sinful, and dangerous, those who were especially powerful—the healers, seers, herbalists, and midwives—were branded witches and were tortured, hung, or burned at the stake. The *Malleus Maleficarum*, handbook of the Inquisition, says outright, "No one does more harm to the Catholic Church than do the midwives." Here is a crucial part of history of which most of us are unaware: the holocaust of women. Estimates of the number of women who died at this time range from several hundred thousand to as many as six million. Not only did the condemned take with them a wealth of healing wisdom passed strictly by oral tradition, but their daughters and sons were forced to witness their silencing, suffering, and death. No wonder we have so much fear of women's power and embodied wisdom—it is encoded in our memories by acts of violence against our female ancestors.

And this is just European and American history. The repression of women's knowledge and power has occurred worldwide, as a result of both religious beliefs and economic factors. As capitalism forged the nuclear family, women were isolated from their kin and were forced to depend on their husbands for financial support in order to raise their young. Thus women lost their tribal ways of jointly raising children, sharing their resources, and pooling their skills. Even the extended family has largely fallen by the wayside, leaving most women entirely on their own to cope with household responsibilities. If we mix in a little religious dogma—that women trick and seduce men, divert their attention from what's important, are dangerous or a mixed blessing at best—we have a recipe for the loss of women's strength and passion.

Think about the gender myths you assimilated in childhood. Consider the overt and covert messages from the media that constantly bombard and envelop us. We've all encoded core beliefs that the feminine spells trouble through "bad girl" characters of the troublemaker, the slut, and the fatal attractor. But the media also portray an opposite ideal of women as loving, giving, virtuous, and self-sacrificing. This is the Madonna/Whore dichotomy, set to derail any attempt at sexual holism. "Good girls" don't want sex as much as men do, but they submit for security's sake, for the sake of home and family. "Bad girls" don't care about security; they are home wreckers and use sex, seduction, and trickery to tame and subdue their male counterparts. Thus, sex becomes a battleground: Men win by domination or evasiveness; women win by calculation or by being "nice."

Not much of a sexual-social legacy, is it? These suppositions are dehumanizing and demeaning to both sexes. They shape a definition of sexuality wherein feminine and masculine are mutually exclusive opposites, with men and women perpetually at odds.

Our core values regarding sex are further expressed by language. Many slang words used to describe the sex act are distinctly unpleasant to women because they portray sex as an act of male aggression toward females. These words also imply that sex equals penetration, that the penis and vagina are the primary sex organs. Not only are there few slang words for women's sexual organs, but none are in common use for the clitoris. This key source of sexual pleasure and response is often left undrawn or unlabeled on anatomical sketches; girls learn the word *clitoris* much later than boys learn the word *penis.* Nancy Friday calls this tantamount to "mental clitoridectomy."[1] Natalie Angier similarly notes that in her research over a five-year period, reference searches in MEDLINE brought up no more than sixty references to the clitoris, as compared to almost thirty times that for the penis.[2]

With regard to sexual activity, male response is the standard against which female response is evaluated and judged. When the penis is suffused with blood, we call it *erect,* but the clitoris is termed *congested.* Even the word *vagina* comes from the Latin for sheath or scabbard, suggesting a waiting and passive receptacle for the penis. As Sheila Kitzinger, beloved authority on childbirth and women's sexuality, astutely observes, "Language is either silent about women's bodies and sexuality or condemns them."[3]

Contraceptive technology played a significant role in loosening sexual mores, as the Pill created new possibilities for sexual experimentation and abortion became more readily available than ever before. Never in history had consumers under the age of thirty dominated the market as they did in the 1960s. This was an era of deep idealism, bright optimism, misguided fanaticism, and genuine courage. This "sexual revolution" seemed promising at first, but in the end, it had very different outcomes for the sexes. Women had more opportunity to express themselves sexually but no longer had a legitimate reason to say "no." Men, on the other hand, had the opportunity to have sex more freely than before without having to take responsibility. In retrospect, the outcome was even greater pressure on women, for although they were free to have sex according to their passions, those who chose not to were labeled inhibited, cold, or even frigid. Cultural beliefs regarding male superiority and privilege remained unaltered, and women felt more enslaved by their sexuality than liberated to its full potential. Many learned the hard way that casual sex seldom engenders intimacy and may actually curtail any possibility of its development.

Even now, when I listen to popular music, I hear messages to the effect that girls are supposed to "put out" sexually, handle the wild and irresponsible behavior of their partners, and somehow cope with their own emotional responses. They must also worry about sexually transmitted infections, pregnancy, and economic dependency should they conceive. Doesn't sound much like liberation to me!

Underlying this polarization of the sexes is the aforementioned disharmony of the masculine and feminine within each of us. Regardless of gender, we all have aggressive, coolly analytical qualities traditionally considered male as well as sensitive, spontaneous qualities traditionally considered female. As we contemplate ways to harmoniously blend these aspects within ourselves, we might also question what makes men and women unique.

Groundbreaking research on this subject was published by Masters and Johnson in 1966, which revealed for the first time women's orgasmic potential and the importance of clitoral stimulation.[4] *Foreplay* became a household word, and although many women still feel that they don't get enough, at least they don't have to explain the term to their partners (although they may need to give detailed instructions). Some feel the term *foreplay* is itself problematic, as it implies that anything short of penetration is merely preliminary and therefore less significant.

But women's need for foreplay can serve as a focal point for appreciating a fundamental difference between the sexes. Although the vast majority of women report that foreplay is important physically, an even greater margin emphasizes the emotional benefits of feeling cared for. When foreplay occurs in a spirit of love and tenderness, it enhances physical relaxation and focus. Without this emotional component, foreplay may feel more irritating than stimulating. This brings to mind the classic dichotomy of male versus female readiness for intimacy: Men need to have sex in order to feel close, while women need to feel close in order to have sex.

How much of this is cultural and how much is biological? Certainly, as primary caretakers of society and its offspring, women need support, particularly in caring for the very young. In our culture, men have traditionally provided the trappings of security. But matrilineal societies still exist where land and possessions are handed down through the woman's line, and women care collectively for one another and the children. These women are closely bonded and protective of each other. This was even more the case in pre-Christian times, when conception was thought to take place by virtue of a woman's relationship to the spirit world. Because men were not considered integral to conception, women did not know or care who fathered their children and so were free of the yoke of male ownership. Notably, these were peaceful cultures, with a strong spiritual orientation.[4]

It took men many thousands of years to perfect the weaponry and warfare necessary to challenge the creative power of the mothers.[5] Eventually, they exerted dominance over women as they did over one another. With the shift to land ownership, women were soon little more than personal property and became dependent on men for survival. Long before the Spanish Inquisition took place, women's innate capacity to heal by way of nature was usurped by men's penchant for tools and instruments.

No one really knows what female sexuality was like before cultural oppression, but we can speculate. The missionary position was probably not the first choice; perhaps women straddled their male consorts, controlling the rate and depth of penetration, generating their own foreplay. According to ancient Tantric traditions (highly reverent of women), the ideal posture of choice was entwined sitting, which allowed a slow, steady buildup of passion that could at the same time be controlled and maintained.

In any case, today we have a complex situation in which traditions of male dominance have been challenged by social upheaval. Women are no longer expected to stay at home and care for their families; they have moved fully into the workforce. Yet many have been disillusioned by the stress and strain of trying to juggle diverse roles of mother, lover, homemaker, and professional. Meanwhile, our economy has so fully adjusted to the two-income family that staying home or cutting back work hours is no longer an option for most. It would seem that women are once again trapped, doomed to overwork or to dependency on men.

Except that men, too, are eager for change. This is the new generation of fathers who have comforted crying babies in the night, changed diapers, and altered their work schedules to take care of sick children. Having done so, many have found the fast track less than appealing and want off. Numerous articles and news polls report that up to 70 percent of women and 40 percent of men would cut back work hours to spend more time with their families, if given the choice. This desire for increased personal time reflects our growing awareness of ebb and flow in the life cycle—we all have times of productivity and exhaustion, creative spurts and phases of dormancy, emotional ups and downs. Despite media images to the contrary, no one is perpetually active and on the go, nor should we try to be. It is no wonder that stress-related illnesses—heart disease, high blood pressure, and eating disorders—plague our society. We desperately need downtime to appreciate and enjoy life, to reconnect with our deepest passions and dreams.

How does this relate to sexuality? As the stereotypical roles of man as aggressive provider and woman as passive caretaker are outmoded, new concepts emerge of male and female needs and desires. This is true not only in the United States; even the most repressive cultures feel the winds of change. For example, a growing number of women activists now speak out against female circumcision. This represents a global shift in values.

I am reminded of a pregnancy and birth video produced in the Netherlands, with a strikingly unusual opening sequence. There was a prolonged shot of a young couple cuddling in bed in the morning, he with his eyes closed, a smile on his face, she talking a bit and nuzzling against his cheek. Sounds like afterglow, but no, this was the tender moment when she broke the news that she was pregnant. What struck me was that here were two equals, both of them vulnerable and strong, in touch with themselves, relaxed and communicative. To her news he responded positively, maturely, with none of that feigned idiot shock the American male typically expresses in our media upon hearing that he is going to be a father. The difference is undoubtedly due in large part to the fact that Holland provides both maternity and paternity leave, home nursing and housekeeping after the baby comes, and generous support, both social and financial, for the developing family.

Separating mind and body, denying the sensual as sacred, leads to a somewhat crude and potentially dangerous definition of sexuality. Apart from the general controversy on the subject, pornography in America must be noted for its unusual violence and brutality. When people are taught to mistrust their bodies and feelings, it's no wonder that their sexual imagery reflects that violation.

We can trace this alienation back to the Garden of Eden myth, wherein Eve made the grievous mistake of commingling with the serpent. In spiritual traditions that predate this myth, the serpent is Kundalini, the vital power of ecstasy that rises up the spine and through the top of the head when sexual energy is united with higher intelligence. My favorite T-shirt message sums it up quite nicely: "Eve Chose Consciousness." She also chose to remember her place in nature, in the circle of life. Yet to this day, most Christian religions maintain that to seek enlightenment through the body is tantamount to sin. What does this mean for women, who have no choice but to unite with their bodies in menstruation, birth, and menopause? What does this mean for all of us but neurosis, isolation, and disease? To quote author, playwright, and poet Susan Griffin:

> *Consciousness and meaning are part of nature.... When bodily knowledge and language are separated, we ourselves experience a terrible separation that ranges all the way from grief to despair to madness.... In this way culture destroys a woman's conscious knowledge of her own experience. Just as she is separated from other women, from her body and her feelings, she is, finally, a stranger to herself.*[6]

Yet, against all odds, women are actively reengaging their natural strengths and unique abilities, their propensities apart from men. They are pulling together in circles, purging themselves of mistrust and competitiveness. They are formulating new communication systems, devising social structures to support them in various life phases, reanimating ritual celebrations from the past, or inventing new ones to suit their needs. Third-wave feminism, highly personal yet imminently practical, springs from our need to unite mind and body, to reclaim our Blood Mysteries as self-affirming and significant events from which we derive great power.

Beyond simply acknowledging that our desire for sex depends on our moods, which fluctuate with both biological and social influences, lies the potential to join with our rhythms instead of working against them, to stop denying the peaks and valleys of our existence and start using them to enhance the quality of our lives, not only for ourselves but also for our loved ones, our culture, our world. To do so is crucial to our survival. To my mind, woman's reunion with her body is a recipe for healing our planetary ills.

Accordingly, we must expand our definition of sexuality to reflect the interrelatedness of all life. We are accustomed to thinking of sexuality in the most limited way, as the physical act alone. A more meaningful and pertinent definition for women is so broad as to be nearly unrecognizable: Sexuality is all that it means to be female, body and soul. This may include physical, erotic expression, but it definitely involves the relationship of our vital energies to other aspects of existence. Actually, the *Webster's* definition is not far off the mark: "The sum of structural, functional and behavioral peculiarities of living beings that subserve reproduction and distinguish males from females."[7]

Let us more closely examine these "behavioral peculiarities" that distinguish women from men. To what extent might these be biologically based? The data show that numerous gender-specific characteristics reveal themselves in early infancy, long before acculturation takes place. For example, baby boys demonstrate a much stronger attraction toward tangible objects than do girls, who are more interested in communication and the human face. Men have better distance vision, but women literally see the big picture: We have wider peripheral vision due to extra rods and cones at the back of the retina. And when it comes to tactile sensitivity, even the least sensitive woman is more sensitive than the most sensitive man.[8]

At the root of these gender-specific traits are differences in brain structure and function that further distinguish the sexes. This is new information for the general public but old news to neuroscientists. For many years, funding was unavailable for research in this area, so pervasive was the belief that cultural influences were the last word in character development. And there was also legitimate concern on the part of female researchers that the data might be used to argue male superiority. But the social and sexual problems cited thus far underscore the need for this information.

In 1990 Susan Faludi made waves with her book *Backlash: The Undeclared War Against American Women*, by documenting how commonly the data has been used to undermine women's gains and accomplishments. To some extent, she perpetuated a feminism that took its aim at men, one that called for sweeping changes in male values and behavior. Then Camille Paglia, author of *Sexual Personae*, declared this sort of feminism self-indulgent and simplistic, fraught with unrealistic expectations of what men must do in order for women to find equality. "Women will never know who they are until they let men be men," she stated, at the same time deriding feminists as self-pitying whiners who needed to get on with their lives.[9] With this polarization, the promise of female autonomy remained elusive, until neurobiological research was brought to public awareness by such authors as Christiane Northrup, Helen Fisher, and Natalie Angier. These women shared a common passion to define women on their own terms, rather than in relationship to men. They placed emphasis on what is right with women, rather than what is wrong with men, thus diffusing some of feminism's excesses and mistaken assumptions. They agreed that patriarchy is a problem, but men are not the target.

To return to the research on brain structure: The fetus produces hormones at about six weeks' gestation that differentiate the sex organs and affect brain development. In 50 percent of females, the prefrontal cortex becomes thicker than it does in males. The cortex contains control centers that govern behavior: In males, functions are highly specialized, or "lateralized" according to hemisphere, but in females, functions are diffused, replicated on both left and right sides of the brain. An outstanding example is that of the emotional centers, which in women are found in both hemispheres but in men are located on the right side only. Add to this the fact that men have verbal centers only in the left hemisphere, and we see a biological basis for the difficulty men may have in expressing their feelings.[10]

Most men show a decided preference for the left side of the brain—associated with linear thinking—whereas women regularly access both hemispheres. Since the right side of the brain has more connections with the body than does the left, women have more access to the body-based wisdom when thinking and speaking than do men.[11]

Women's ability to switch easily from one side of the brain to the other results from an enlargement of the parts of the brain that connect the two hemispheres—the corpus callosum and the anterior commissure.[12] This may explain women's ability to handle several tasks simultaneously, while men prefer to focus on one thing at a time. Women's attention is generally more diffused and multifaceted than men's. Thus our approach to problem solving is to encircle, to consider a problem from a variety of angles before distilling a solution. Men tend to break down and categorize as they solve problems, adding up factors methodically, bricklayer-style. This is why, when the sexes try to solve problems together, men are at a loss to understand why women bring in so many seemingly unrelated factors and can't get to the point, while women wonder why men must be so controlling and tight-lipped—what's wrong with talking things through? Women by nature tend to expand, while men contract.

We can readily extrapolate these tendencies to discrepancies in sexual needs. In his groundbreaking book *Men, Women and Relationships,* John Gray suggests that a basic misunderstanding of ignorance of key differences between the sexes is at the root of most sexual unhappiness and dysfunction. What does a woman need from a lover? Assistance in focusing! Especially after a busy day, she needs help bringing her diffused and expanded awareness back to herself and her body. It has been shown that women need an average of eighteen minutes of stimulation to reach orgasm, whereas men need only two or three.[13] Women need cuddling; they need to be touched in a nonsexual way at first, erogenous zones aside.

Gray further observes that the delicious, total-body pleasure felt by women with this warm-up is usually experienced by men only after they climax, because men tend to focus and contract their sexual

tension until they ejaculate. Both sexes can help each other by recognizing and balancing their differences; he, by taking the time to
help his partner relax, she, by making the wait enjoyable for him or
by being up for an occasional "quickie."

But apart from our relationships with men, we women have our
own inherent mechanisms for growth and exploration: our biological rhythms. The monthly cycle moves us through an exquisite sequence of moods and passions: Each time around, we experience
the spectrum. Menstruation is the *petite morte,* the end of one cycle
and the beginning of another, when we have opportunity to reflect
on lingering disappointments and frustrations in our lives, letting
them go or seeking resolution. Menstruation also links us to the
rhythms of the moon, which profoundly influence our existence.
Later, when we no longer have need of the monthly cycle because
we have learned its lessons through and through, we cease menstruating and retain our "wise blood" for the benefit of society. These
biological imperatives give our lives meaning; they are vehicles for
transformation.

Yet all of this may be negatively affected by our culture's determi-
nation to keep us in a caretaking role. Women do have some biological predilection to nurture, but this has been grossly exploited by
society. Remember that in patriarchal systems such as ours, women
are subordinate and are held responsible to men before themselves.
Thus scientific evidence of hormonal prompts for maternal behavior has been used against women as a gauge of femininity, despite
the fact that there is no indication that these nurturing behaviors
extend in any significant degree to the care of grown men, let alone
those outside the immediate family.

Nevertheless, women have for generations been made to live
their lives through others. Their worth has been contingent on how
well they foster male superiors: "Behind every good man, there's a
good woman." If there are problems in the family, guilt and blame
invariably fall on the woman. She is responsible for making it work:
discerning problems, implementing solutions, and blending every-

thing in perfect harmony. Predictably, this task consumes whatever time she might otherwise find for herself. And how is she expected to respond to this pressure? She is to be self-sacrificing, stoic, faithful, and complacent to life's "realities," yet willing and able to fight fiercely for her kin. Though ludicrous to many of us today, the social construct persists.

If we nurture others to the exclusion of ourselves, we attempt to live out our dreams and desires through them as well. As the contemporary saying reminds us, "Women marry hoping to change their partners; men marry hoping their partners will never change." We must, once and for all, see this for what it is: a recipe for loss and disappointment. Only by establishing our own needs and goals as priorities can we hope to find fulfillment in life. Although we may nurture and care for others to some extent, let this be by choice rather than by obligation.

In light of all this, it is hardly surprising that although women are better educated and more sophisticated now than at any time in recent history, we remain puzzled by and thus at the mercy of our biological rhythms, unable to incorporate them into our lives. This is largely because these rhythms engender an ebb-and-flow approach to living distinctly at odds with the male "ladder of success" model. But the time has come for us to share with our partners and society a truer definition of what it means to be a woman. These are the things women know: that everything comes around, that reflection is germane to creative action, and that the passage of time alone can be a key factor in change. We have learned these things organically through the monthly cycle, in gestating our young, in weathering the stages of marriage and child rearing, in transforming through menopause. As society cries out for balance, for solutions to pressing crises in health care, education, and the environment, women's wisdom is once again coming to the fore. Women are speaking out, acting up, and making the difference.

CHAPTER 2

Sexual Awakening

When was your first experience of sexual awakening? Not necessarily your first sexual interaction, but your own experience of coming alive to your sexual nature?

This may be a bit hard to pin down because sexuality is with us from birth. Even as infants, we are saturated with the "love hormone," *oxytocin,* when breast-feeding. One woman compared her first orgasm to the feeling of ecstasy and physical release she experienced when walking through puddles as a child. Some of us remember the first time we touched ourselves sexually, or perhaps were touched by another in a spirit of play and exploration.

The first time I can ever recall having a feeling of what society calls arousal is when I was about four years old. I would use the palm of my hand and roll it up into a fist and sit on it and rub back and forth until I had an orgasm. Sometimes I would use a towel, a blanket or anything that was around me. When I was five years old, my twelve-year-old brother caught me "wiggling" (that's what he called it) and said he was going to tell my mom and that I was going to be in big trouble. I was ashamed and embarrassed that he caught me, and I really didn't want my mother to know what I had been doing. A few days later my mom and I were on a walk and she asked me if I knew what the terms wiggling or humping meant. Of course, I denied everything.

I was in the fifth grade now and still humping and wiggling. I was constantly aroused, it seemed. Whatever I was doing, I knew I had this little secret that could make me feel so good inside, and I always wanted to use it. It never mattered when those feelings came on. If I was in school, I would get a hall pass to go to the bathroom and would wait until no one was in there, then I would get on the floor and sit on my hands until I felt great.

Masturbation is with us from a very early age. Books on child care typically reassure parents not to worry if their one-year-old son plays frequently with his penis, or their baby daughter often has her hand between her legs. But if the hormones associated with sexual maturation and the sex drive are not present to a significant degree, why does this happen? Again, the answer is oxytocin. This hormone is released not only with direct genital contact but also at the mere thought of physical pleasure. Oxytocin has been called the love hormone because it engenders feelings of desire, tenderness, affection, and intimacy.

Billy Adams touched me. I'll never forget it! I was very young, maybe seven years old. We locked ourselves in the bathroom and played doctor. He examined me. It's all sort of a blur in my memory except the moment when he touched me. I had never felt anything before that brought me so into the present and opened me up to my place in nature all in the same instant. Unfortunately, that moment was cut short. We were discovered just as he was touching me and he was sent home. We were not allowed to play together anymore. Too bad. I could have learned a lot about myself and my body right then in a very sweet and innocent way.

From then on, I kept feelings of where I fit in nature very private, thinking they were wrong and bad. I always thought there was something wrong with me for thinking about my place in nature and my body as just a part of it, the same as a dog or raccoon.

In spite of the naturalness of our promptings, many of us are made to feel guilty and ashamed by our first sexual impulses. This is particularly true of girls, whose parents feel they must do whatever possible to keep them from getting interested in sex too soon lest unplanned pregnancy occur. Nevertheless, curiosity about sex happens when it will, often at a much earlier age than sex-ed programs in the schools reflect.

My sexuality was shaped greatly by the era I grew up in. My mother was a flower child, a hippie; the sexual revolution was still in full effect in her life. I was raised in a communal situation for the first six years of my life, and I think I must have witnessed some sexual affection between my parents or their friends—it would have been pretty difficult not to, living and traveling in a school bus together up the West Coast! I have hazy memories of hearing my mom make noises with my dad that I now know to be sex/pleasure sounds. I was definitely curious as to what they were doing, and I can remember calling out and asking them one particular night.

Later on, I remember being in the third or fourth grade, sneaking into the living room to watch TV in the middle of the night, turning it down so low I had to strain to hear the dialogue. We had cable, and I found Lady Chatterly's Lover *on Showtime. My whole body knew this was a movie I should not be watching, but I had to see it through. That was the first time I had ever really seen sex. The movie sent feelings through my body that I had no clue what to do with. This was what everyone did in their bedroom?*

And another account:

My sexuality was completely formed by society, TV, magazines, and older friends. Even when I did not know what sex was, I knew it had to do with males and females being close and comfortable with each other. When I think back to what I first thought about sex, I thought it had nothing to do with the woman's pleasure, it was purely to satisfy the man, and women just had to do it in order to be loved.

After many questions and much research, I discovered it had something to do with the vagina and the penis. Even at the age of six or seven I was able to put two and two together and figure out that if a man could do it, I most definitely could do it by myself. So one night I explored. I remember feeling funny, but I kept telling myself, "It's your body, you shouldn't feel funny touching it." That was the night I discovered my very own sexuality.

From these accounts, we can surmise that girls become sexually awakened at quite a young age, and that most would appreciate clear and accurate information on the subject much sooner than we tend to provide it. It is also poignantly evident that for us to impart a sense of guilt or shame to a girl regarding her sexual behavior can have a devastating effect on her self-esteem. She can stop neither her sexual drives nor her sexual curiosity, but if she learns to associate these impulses with wrongdoing, her opinion of herself will inevitably decline. Recall from Chapter 1 women's contextual, relational tendencies in learning, in life—much more so than boys, girls take to heart the feelings and opinions of others.

This brings to mind the wonderful work of Carol Gilligan, and her book *In a Different Voice*. In her research, Gilligan found that girls reach a critical point around the age of nine or ten when they begin to doubt their natural instincts and abilities. As a result, they lose their "voice"; that is, their ability to speak up for themselves and maintain their own opinions.[1] Interestingly enough, this is not as contemporary a phenomenon as we might think but dates back to at least the early 1900s.

Why is this so? Remember that girls develop differently than boys. Even at birth, the brains of each differ in structure and function. In boys, the left hemisphere of the cortex tends to develop much more rapidly than in girls, who have relatively equal development in both hemispheres. In other words, girls have an inherent balance of the nonlinear, intuitive aspects of the right hemisphere and the linear, logical aspects of the left hemisphere.[2] When given aptitude tests on ethical decision making, girls tend to score lower than boys precisely because they see the big picture, bringing in so many variables that their answers are considered too vague to score. This contextual, relational way of thinking comes naturally to girls, but when they realize it is not valued by our society, they either quiet down or just give up.[3] As we try to support our daughters and help them mature, it is crucial that we teach them to resist this culturally based oppression, lest it turn into suppression of their own instinctive wisdom. How can we do this? Notice that the age at which girls tend to lose their voices dovetails with the average age of menarche (the first menstruation). This is more than a coincidence. As is true of all the Blood Mysteries, the period leading up to the main event is charged with emotion, chaos, uncertainty; in approaching menarche, girls typically become uppity and outspoken. This is a grand opportunity for us to witness and stand by supportively, encouraging their candor and forthrightness. Many cultures formalize this major life transition with ceremony and celebration. And in most such ceremonies, women of all ages welcome the young woman into the community at large. The following are ideas on how to develop a Menarche Rite.

The Menarche Rite*

Women have definite physiologic milestones that herald major life transitions. There was a time when these transitions were held holy, and served to connect us with the rhythms and cycles of the seasons and the moon. The first of these milestones is the Menarche Initiation Rite, held at the time of a young woman's first menses to honor her crossing from girlhood to womanhood.

(cont'd.)

In the past, it was customary to mark this major change in a woman's life with a special observance or celebration. Anticipation of this honoring helped the girl greet her first bleeding with joy and triumph; it was the most essential of all initiation rites.

In nonindustrial societies, seclusion is a nearly universal component of the menarche rite, not out of fear but in reverence for the sacred power of menstrual blood. In some indigenous cultures, girls are isolated for several years. Young Dyak women of Southeast Asia spend a year in a white cabin, wearing white clothes and eating white foods only (thought to ensure good health).[10] While alone, they contemplate their physical transformation to womanhood and consider what society expects of them. Elder women visit periodically to teach the art and craft of womanhood, including the responsibilities of sexuality and child rearing. This has enormous impact on their personal growth.

One of the most beautiful examples of menarche initiation is the Apache rite of "Changing Woman." In this solemn ceremony, the pubescent girl becomes the primordial Apache mother, "White Painted Woman." She reenacts the story of Changing Woman who, impregnated by the sun, gave birth to the Apache people. On the first day, she is sprinkled with yellow cattail pollen to symbolize fertility and is taught by wise women of the "fire within," her sacred sexuality. The ceremony lasts for four days, in honor of the Four Directions. On the final night, the young woman must dance from sunset to sunrise for the wellbeing of her people. At dawn, this song is sung to her:

Now you are entering the world.
You will become an adult with responsibilities

(cont'd.)

Walk with honor and dignity.
Be strong!
For you are the mother of our people
For you will become the mother of a nation.[11]

Although a four-day ritual may seem excessive in the context of our busy lifestyles, its purpose of enabling young women to experience heightened awareness of their new status and power is highly relevant. Menarche rites of today can range from a formal ceremony to a simple gathering of women friends and relatives for a wonderful meal together: The main idea is to distinguish this milestone event from everyday life. Although some mothers wish to create these ceremonies for their daughters, it is crucial that young women themselves participate in the design and content of their celebrations, choosing what is comfortable for them.

Here are some suggestions for a memorable event. The place where the celebration will be held can be decorated with candles, flowers, or ribbons of red and white, red symbolizing blood and life force, and white representing innocence, strength, and reproductive health. The young woman may wish to sit at the place of honor, the head of the table perhaps, with her chair decorated like a throne. The centerpiece might be of red roses, one for each year she has lived. She may also want to wear a crown of flowers, signifying her flowering womanhood.

To begin, the group can acknowledge and invoke the young woman's family line, all those who have crossed this threshold before. This affirms her place in the community of women, her procreative potential, and the natural beauty of her menarche experience.

The main part of the rite involves sharing information on menstruation through storytelling and first person accounts.

(cont'd.)

Each participant is given the opportunity to describe her menarche experience. Not all of these stories will be joyous; older women may become very emotional if they recall feeling ashamed of their first blood. Yet this creates even stronger intent within the circle to honor the young woman currently in the midst of this Blood Mystery.

An ancient form of honoring menarche is the Clay Rite, similar to the Apache use of cattail pollen. This is only appropriate if the young woman feels comfortable enough to be nude in the presence of her friends. Those who have not yet started bleeding cover her with wet, red clay to symbolize her connection to the earth. This can be fun—a playful, messy act of saying farewell to childhood.

If they are in a rural setting, the group may wish to construct a sweat lodge for the young woman, where she may spend a certain amount of time in seclusion. As an alternative, she might spend a night alone in a tent or cabin with her friends close by, singing or drumming to give her courage. Or she might simply go off by herself to a place of total privacy.

While in solitude, several "wise women" or a special relative may come to her with instructions regarding her fertility and responsibilities in the next stage of life. When they are finished, she can return to the larger group. Her friends may wish to form a birth arch at this point, lining up and passing the young woman through their legs until she finally comes to her mother, who brings her out and into her embrace. As with actual birth, there is a moment in this act where time seems suspended—the power of this ritual is tangible.

The "newborn" woman may then be washed clean of remaining mud by those of her friends who have already begun bleeding, welcoming her into the adult community

(cont'd.)

of women. She should then be dressed in new, beautiful clothing she can treasure for years to come, fussed over, and adorned like the Goddess herself!

The group may then make some final affirmations regarding the power of menstruation and appropriate roles for women to play in today's society. Each participant may also wish to confide her own special ways of honoring her menstrual period. To close, the young woman's mother may give her some jewelry, perhaps a family heirloom piece, or anything featuring red stones. She may also want to formally present her daughter to whatever higher power they recognize, asking for protection and guidance.

When the ritual ends, feasting begins. Red foods represent fertility; guests may wish to toast the young woman with red wine. Perhaps other family members will choose to participate at this point. Men often find it hard to stay away during the ceremony and are very pleased when finally welcomed to join the festivities. Above all, this ritual should be exactly as the young woman wants it, so that she may discover a new degree of trust in her body and in herself.

If such a formal ritual seems too complex or inappropriate for your family, simple variations are fine. One mother told her daughter that when she got her period, she could choose any three things to do in celebration. On the first day of her menarche, she opted for: 1) a shopping trip; 2) total silence from Mom for the entire day; 3) a steak. The last was somewhat controversial for this vegetarian family, but as her mother observed, "Eating a steak was my daughter's ultimate statement of adult decision-making power."

Another option is for mother and daughter to go off together to some favorite outdoor place, connecting with nature and each other. They may go hiking or canoeing, or

(cont'd.)

perhaps build a campfire together, as long as they spend time alone and make it a celebratory day. The mother could use this time to review her daughter's birth and childhood, with stories of what she was like when she was younger, and all the great things she has done in her life thus far. She might also share her visions and her hopes for her daughter's future.

In addition to the aforementioned gift of jewelry, some mothers allow their daughters to pierce their ears on this day, presenting them a gift of earrings with red stones. Another precious keepsake is a "Menarche Book," comprised of photos of all the women in the family (suitable for passing on to the next generation).

The day could end with the mother drawing a bath for her daughter, perhaps placing flower petals on the water. When it is over, the two can decide how to share the news with the rest of the family, and whether a special event of some kind is desired. Again, the most important thing is the young woman's comfort; if she happily participates in planning a larger celebration, she will joyfully remember it for the rest of her life.

Once a girl has reached the age of ten, she becomes increasingly socially identified and needs more than her mother's opinions. Although most girls get their information on sex from TV, the Internet, magazines, movies, and so on, the stories and advice of other female relatives or wise friends could help counterbalance any negative imprints.

In fact, more than any time in recent history, young women are interested in hearing stories from their elders. Storytelling is oral tradition, and as such, bears different meaning from what we read in books: The storyteller is just as much a part of the story as the setting and events. When experienced women tell their young cohorts stories of their own Blood Mystery experiences, they help them to see the continuity of these events reflected in who they are and what they have become.

Returning to menarche for a moment: What is happening to a girl at the physical level? She experiences surges of estrogen, progesterone, and testosterone for many months before levels stabilize sufficiently to initiate menstruation. To experience menarche she must also have enough body fat, at least 17 percent of her total body weight (this is why anorexic, extremely thin, or highly athletic young women often do not menstruate, a condition known as amenorrhea). For sustained menstruation and regular cycles, a young woman needs about 22 percent body fat. Her first cycles may be anovulatory (meaning that no egg is released), but gradually her body will catch on, and her cycle will be established.

The average age of menstruation is creeping downward; it is not uncommon for girls today to experience menarche at age ten. Just a few decades ago, the average was age twelve. What is happening here? It appears that a potent combination of chemical estrogens in our environment and growth-stimulating hormones in dairy/animal products may be causing menarche to occur earlier and earlier (see Chapter 3 for more details). Our girls are literally being forced to grow up before they are emotionally ready. All the more reason for treating menarche as a rite of passage. Consider the following account:

> I remember wanting to get my period because then I'd be a woman and I felt like, wow. I used to go to these meetings with my mom and the older women would talk about it, it was such a common thing that was always talked about. PMS, you know—they'd kid around about it. When my mom's friends bled at the same time, it was like this really bonding thing between them, and I always wanted to be a part of that. And then I got my period—I woke up and I was so excited! I had just started seventh grade, and I felt so much older and wiser.
>
> The Menarche Rite was my mom's idea. She had read about it and brought the idea home to me. At first I didn't want to do it

because it was my own private thing, but then I thought it might be fun. My mom and I talked about it and I read lots of books about it, and then we started to plan the ritual. I was having so much fun with it. I was really excited about this high-mark rite where I could become a woman, and all my closest friends and all the women that had always been closest to me all my life would be there.

We planned it out on note cards. Everybody had different things they would do. We made an altar with family photographs of all the women before me. My mother and I brought flowers. We made another little altar in the middle of the table with tampons and pads all over it and candles—it was so beautiful. I had a beautiful silk dress my mother had gotten for me. I was totally in a daze; I just loved it! It was my ritual! I felt grown up, part of the circle of women.

Now I look at my bleeding as a natural thing and not at all a pain in the ass. Lots of my girlfriends groan and say, "Oh, God, I've got my period," like it's a bad thing. I look at it as such a beautiful thing that millions of women have gone through, and the ritual made me feel that way. I have my menarche box at home with all my stuff in it—I'm really thankful for that.[4]

I strongly believe that a young woman's experience of menarche affects the quality of her first sexual encounter. If her menarche is honored, especially by adult women in a way that also has meaning to her, she is apt to respect her body and herself too much to casually surrender her virginity. Unfortunately, a high percentage of young women have unhappy first experiences.

I really loved this guy, and had certainly had opportunities before to be sexual with others, but for me, he was the one. I was just fifteen, and he was nineteen, already in college. We went off to a friend's beach house, and he fixed me a drink (my first one) and we took a shower together. One thing led to another, and the moment came.

Even though it didn't hurt that much, I guess because I'd already masturbated and had things inside me, I didn't feel much of anything. He actually accused me of not being a virgin, which made me feel awful. He didn't call me for two weeks, and then he was distant. Later, through a friend, I found out he was getting married to someone else. I carried the torch for a while…then gave it up. It was two years before I had sex with anyone else.

Another account:

Starting when I was eight years old, my brothers and I were sent to our grandmother's house for several summers because our mom was sick and couldn't deal with three little kids at the time. We slept in the back room after spending all day at the beach. My oldest brother, who was twelve, would put his hand or his mouth under the covers at night and play with me. I liked the feeling, but felt very naughty for liking and wanting it. Because of this conflict, I felt paralyzed and didn't do anything, I just lay there and let him do want he wanted to me. That feeling of paralysis—not being able to say what I want and don't want—left me feeling powerless.

My brother's desire for me escalated as he grew into his teens. I began to feel that the only way to be liked by a man was to give him whatever he wanted of my body.

This account not only is disturbing but also crosses the line into incest. Yet many young women report first sexual encounters with older brothers. Where are their mothers, why can't they tell them, and why aren't their mothers aware?

And another, equally distressing:

When I was seventeen I had been dating a boy for three months, and he wanted to know how much longer I was going to hold out before giving it to him. I wasn't sure I wanted to take my pants off, and why should I? I knew I could make myself feel great just by kissing and rubbing back and forth on his penis through my clothes. He said that caused him great pain and that if I thought that felt great, just wait until the real thing. I was scared. I did love him and I didn't want him to leave just 'cause I wouldn't take my pants off.

One week later I gave it up to him, and it was nothing like the great secret I had of making myself feel good. I was in a lot of pain, there was bleeding, there were tears, and there was no orgasm. I was thoroughly disappointed with him, with society, and with myself for giving up something that was so special to me for ninety seconds of sheer terror.

Why are these initial experiences so often unsatisfying? If a woman is partnered with a young man, he will often rush to intercourse without adequate foreplay. As Theresa Crenshaw points out in her book *The Alchemy of Lust*, sexual exploration just shy of intercourse invariably involves lots of kissing, holding, petting, and fondling, which serve to dramatically increase oxytocin levels in both partners. When this prolonged period of foreplay is either replaced by intercourse or cut short, women in particular miss the closeness and pleasure engendered by high levels of oxytocin.[5]

They may also miss orgasm altogether. According to a study conducted at the University of Chicago involving three thousand women aged eighteen to thirty-nine, 25 percent were unable to achieve orgasm during intercourse.

Psychologist Alfred Ells, author of the book *Restoring Innocence,* observes that first sexual experiences have tremendous power to imprint us either for good or ill. In this case, imprinting refers to a process of deeply internalizing the attitudes and beliefs of an intimate partner under circumstances of great stress or extreme excitement. Ells believes that first-lover imprints can influence sexual behavior and the capacity for sexual enjoyment for many years to come.

Here is a young woman's story that demonstrates how positive feelings about herself and her body contributed to a wonderful first experience. Although not specifically mentioned, it seems clear that

an open and loving relationship with her mother played a significant part in her ability to wait to have sex until she was truly ready:

*I had my first kiss at age fourteen with my boyfriend. I felt a whole
new arousal in making out with him and had my first orgasm fully
clothed, rubbing our bodies together. We explored each other's
bodies, went skinny-dipping in his pool, and I had my first intense
orgasm during oral sex when we snuck away during a camping
trip with my family. This was the first time I remember feeling
out of control, an out-of-body erotic feeling. Once I started to experience orgasms, I realized I could do it by myself. I found my
mother's vibrator and used it every so often, or the lid from my teen
perfume, Love's Baby Soft.*

*About masturbation, my mother had a talk with me once and
I remember her saying that it was okay to do, it was natural. At
some point, I got influenced by other sources and I would sometimes feel guilty doing it so often. This wore off as I grew older and
formed my own beliefs.*

*I began to feel more sexy. I loved dancing nude in front of the
mirror, I loved the way my body looked and the way the curves
felt. I dated a lot and experimented with guys as much as one can
without having intercourse. During my junior year, I started dating my old boyfriend again. After six months, I decided that even
if he wasn't "the one," I did love him, and I wouldn't regret losing
my virginity to him. We discussed birth control, and I talked to my
mother about it and decided on a diaphragm. I was fitted for one,
and we set a date. A romantic weekend at his parents' cabin, with
gifts and champagne, and he was so gentle that I had an orgasm
that first time.*

This young woman, aged nineteen, also had a positive first experience, and had this to say to other young women hoping to have
the same:

*I think sex is looked on much too lightly in this society, I believe this
to be one of the most detrimental outcomes of our society's way of*

expressing itself in the twenty-first century. Sex is a sacred act that not only invades a woman's body but also makes it very possible that she could be carrying a baby in her belly for the next nine months, labor that baby into the world, and be a mommy for the rest of her life. In my opinion, we should not have any mommies who do not want to be, or are not ready to be, mommies.

As I casually flip through the channels on TV, I am appalled at what I see. I don't think there is one show on TV these days that portrays that it is not only okay, it is a woman's right not to sleep with a man on the first date. Sex should be portrayed as a woman's right, and also as a man's privilege to enter her most sacred temple, her body. On TV, if a woman does decide to open her sacred body to a man she has barely known for two hours, she is not expected to gain much from this experience: She of course will not have an orgasm, but he of course will completely get off.

My heart goes out to all the young girls growing up in our society today, molding their sexuality to what they see on TV, and comparing themselves to these unempowered women, or dolls, I should say, in the magazines. What a hard struggle it will be for them to find their true identity and discover that they're only as unique and beautiful as they make themselves out to be. That their sexuality is their own, and their body, a temple to be entered only by the most sacred individual in their eyes.

How can we reinstill a sense of the sacred into sexuality? I think one of the best ways is to teach young women more about the power and beauty of their bodies at a basic physical level. Old imagery of the female body as a passive vessel for male pleasure must be replaced with new scientific findings that show quite the opposite to be true.

For example, standard explanations of the process of conception purport that the egg is passive, almost stupid, indiscriminately waiting to be penetrated by whatever sperm comes along. But observations by fiber optics show the egg to be quite selective, chemically rejecting a considerable number of sperm until finally permitting one to come inside:

> *That thick, extracellular coat [of the egg] is the famed zona pellu-cida—the translucent zone—the closest thing a mammalian egg has to a shell. The zona pellucida is a thick matrix of sugar and protein that is as cunning as a magnetic field. It invites sperm to explore its contours, but then repels what doesn't suit it. It decides who is friend and who is alien.*[6]

The cervix also plays an active role in conception only recently revealed by fiber optics. Quite the opposite of the immobile, passive organ we once envisioned it to be, it actually dips up and down as the uterus contracts during orgasm. In this, there is a link to a woman's chance of conceiving. If her partner ejaculates and she orgasms soon after, her cervix will dip repeatedly into seminal fluid pooled at the end of her vagina, drawing it up inside her. Timing is everything, and the cervix actively participates.[7] And apparently, there are more than emotional factors involved when a woman whose partner has already climaxed decides to "go for it" herself.

Young women also need a deeper understanding of the role of the clitoris in pleasure and orgasm. The clitoral system, although embedded within the pelvis, has as much or more erectile tissue than the male penis. However, the clitoris lacks a venous plexus, which in men prevents blood from flowing out of the aroused penis. In women, blood flow in and out of the aroused clitoris is flexible and fairly continuous, which makes it more adaptable to varying degrees of stimulation, able to distend and relax quickly. This accounts for women's marvelous ability to have multiple orgasms during a single sexual encounter.[8]

Last but not least, women need a better understanding of the vagina: how it is strong, how it is vulnerable. As Natalie Angier brightly declares, "The vagina is its own ecosystem, a land of unsung symbiosis and tart vigor."[9] Women everywhere are still taught that the vagina is dirty, but it is actually quite clean—cleaner than the mouth. Yes, the vagina is full of bacteria, but they are healthy lacto-bacilli organisms (like those found in yogurt) that literally eat back offending types. Normal vaginal discharge is just that—normal. It is composed of the same ingredients as blood serum (what is left in blood when the red cells are separated out).

What causes vaginal infection? Ironically, a major cause is douching. This practice, which is supposed to leave us feeling "clean and fresh," actually puts us at risk by washing away those friendly lactobacilli we need for vaginal health. For a heterosexual woman who has not been active for a while, another source of vaginal infection may be seminal fluid (healthy, no STIs). Vaginal pH is normally quite acidic, around 3.8 to 4.5, while seminal fluid is alkaline, with a pH around 8. For the vagina unused to it, exposure to seminal fluid can cause an overgrowth of yeast organisms normally present in limited amounts (there may also be an immunological reaction to a new partner's sperm, if only at first).

Returning to the theme of masturbation, it is vitally important that every young woman realize the freedom and pleasure to be had in this harmless practice. As a society, we don't frown on masturbation, but we don't exactly condone it. Yet it is a clear alternative for women not yet ready to be sexually active, or for those taking a sexual time-out.

My sexual coming of age was sort of a "group effort." My house-mate's boyfriend bought her the book Sex for One, *by Betty Dodson, and it soon made its way around the house. We were all in our late teens or early twenties and had experimented with masturbation, but Betty opened our eyes to a whole new sexual arena: the vibrator.*

I remember the first night I used it. Taking the advice of good ol' Betty, I took a bath to relax, because I knew I had an audience in the other room waiting for a rave review. Even though I had masturbated before, I had never had an orgasm, and I really didn't expect to have one right away. Several months later, I actually did.

I was blown away, to say the least. It made me so happy to know that I didn't have to depend on another person for sexual satisfaction. Since I was the only one of my friends that was still a virgin, I was beginning to think my sex life would never get off the ground. Using the vibrator totally changed all that. I especially liked knowing that in the blink of an eye I could run up to my room and get myself off. No one could stop me, and I didn't need anyone to help me either. My sexuality was mine now. I felt like I held a great power that women have not tapped into, for whatever reason.

Knowing that my sexuality is mine, I view sex a bit differently. I still feel it is something to be held sacred between those involved. But now, knowing the power I feel in my own sexuality, I want to share it. I feel more comfortable being intimate with others, maybe because I don't play mind games with myself as I used to, or maybe because I am so much more mature than I used to be.

Self-discovery, self-affirmation, and self-respect are the cornerstones of a young woman's sexual maturation. Even if she has a rocky start with menarche or her first love is a disappointment, she can still find her way, especially with the help of other women. Here is a story of one woman's transformation:

The stories I heard in quiet corners with hushed voices were horror stories about how each woman in our family was handling the "curse." It was clear from the beginning that having your period was not anything to be happy about. I was given detailed instructions on how to deal with this "menace," for if I did not, I would suffer greatly like those before me. Cramps, bloating, huge blood loss, headaches, fainting spells—the list went on and on.

For the next seven years I popped pills, made sure every tampon was deodorized, and kept constant vigilance on my calendar lest some fun activity present itself when I was expecting to bleed. Needless to say, this behavior of self-abhorrence left its mark on my relationships. I completely denied my feminine self, and wanted to be one of the guys. I was built athletically and was highly competitive, and I considered most women to be weak, "frilly," and only concerned with "simple" things.

What I didn't understand until much later was that because I had rejected my biology and my femininity, my relationships with men would be little more than a reflection of my self-loathing. If I couldn't enjoy my body as a woman, I couldn't enjoy sex—although I thought I was at the time. Basically, though, I was there to please. Not even thinking that I had desires. Men were the ones who needed sex; I just played along.

After several years of falling and getting back up again, I am aware of the deep-seated hatred I had for women. I especially disliked women who enjoyed the arts of cooking, sewing, baking, and child rearing. Women who were vulnerable, loving, and open to truly experience life would push my buttons and make me really uncomfortable. Then, after I had my son, I came to realize that deep down in me was that woman—I love to cook, bake, be with my son, love deeply, garden, sculpt, and paint. My cycle took on a whole new meaning for me. I started wearing natural cotton menstrual pads instead of tampons, saving my blood in a menstrual bowl and giving it back to the earth. I'd take the entire first day of my flow and do whatever felt right, holding it as a sacred time in my life. I changed my viewpoint and also my words—words have power. I now practice the art of fertility awareness. I touch and smell my body daily; it is a temple to me now.

As I was starting these practices, I noticed a shift in my perception of other women. No longer would I walk down the street and try to make eye contact with a man who was walking with another women. Instead, I made eye contact with her. I grew to love women, because I was growing to love myself.

In the next chapter, we will learn more about how women are reclaiming the menstrual cycle, including the sexual peaks it engenders.

CHAPTER 3

Dancing *with* Our Hormones

Sometime in my early twenties, I remember wondering why female animals went into heat while women apparently did not. Why would this universal fact of mammalian sexuality be omitted from the most highly evolved species? Scientists have conjectured that the intellectual aspect of human desire long ago preempted any underlying biological patterns. Yet this did not explain my own fluctuations of desire, seemingly unrelated to person, mood, or setting. Lacking any leads for the time being, I put my question on hold.

The turning point in my inquiry came after the birth of my second child. It was time to resume birth control, and having tried almost every method available with minimal satisfaction, I chose to learn fertility awareness. I soon discovered why postpartum women are often discouraged in this pursuit. Because I was breast-feeding and not yet menstruating, my hormone levels fluctuated frequently, and my fertility signals were all over the spectrum. But after months of observation, I began to catch on. Once I reestablished my cycle, I observed my signs and symptoms of fertility not only in mucus changes and basal temperature fluctuations but also in the sexual mood swings that accompanied these. Beyond a doubt, I saw that my desire for sex was greater when I was fertile. I also noticed that I made copious amounts of slippery secretion midcycle, which made lovemaking easy and seemed to stimulate my partner and me with its distinctive, erotic scent. Perhaps, I thought, we women have a "heat" of our own after all!

I recall attending a midwifery conference some years ago, when a physician (one of the few male presenters) mentioned in passing that according to his patients, the ovulatory phase was the time they felt most like making love. "How about the only time!" one of the women in the audience piped up, and the entire room broke into laughter. A moment of truth, it seems, and in marked contrast to the "anytime, ever-ready" notion perpetuated by the media.

Since then, numerous studies have focused on women's hormones and how they affect health, personality, behavior, and sexual response. Let's look at these key hormones, considering their actions in detail, and then we can explore the delicate choreography of their effects within the monthly cycle.

The Hormones

What, exactly, are hormones? The word *hormone* comes from the Greek *horman*, which means to arouse, excite. Hormones are secreted by certain tissues in the body and travel via the blood or other fluids to other tissues, which they stimulate in particular ways. We used to think there was a difference between hormones and neurotransmitters—the chemicals that allow brain cells to communicate—but now we know that hormones also trigger activity in the brain.

Even more interesting is the fact that hormones are not nearly as specific in origin as we once thought. For example, *estrogen* (considered the quintessential female hormone) is made primarily by the ovaries under signals from the pituitary gland, which is regulated by the hypothalamus. However, estrogen is also made and utilized by the bones and the blood.

Estrogen plays a major role during puberty, causing breast development, changes in sweat glands that produce body odor, changes in the vagina and its secretions, and enlargement of the external genitals (the labia and clitoris). In a sexually mature woman, estrogen triggers ovulation, and during pregnancy it is responsible for breast growth, vaginal and cervical changes, and uterine enlargement.

Progesterone is another key hormone in women's lives. It is produced by the ovaries, specifically by the disintegrated egg follicle known as the corpus luteum. Once ovulation has occurred, progesterone keeps the uterine lining growing so that it can sustain the embryo in the event of conception. During pregnancy, it reduces uterine irritability so the uterus will retain its contents. Eventually, the placenta takes charge of its manufacture.

Now let's see how these hormones work in concert during an average cycle of twenty-eight days. On day one, as menstruation begins, one of the pituitary hormones, *follicle-stimulating hormone (FSH)*, begins to surge. It triggers the ovaries to start producing estrogen, which, around day five, enters the bloodstream and flows to the pituitary gland. When estrogen reaches a certain level, the pituitary secretes less FSH and releases another hormone, *luteinizing hormone (LH)*.

This brings us to midcycle, or day fourteen. Estrogen is at its peak, and LH flows to the ovary to stimulate one of the follicles there to ripen and release an egg. The egg bursts from the follicle and is drawn into the fallopian tube: This is ovulation. Once empty, the follicle becomes the corpus luteum and starts to produce progesterone.

Please refer to the diagram on the next page. Note that estrogen levels peak mid-month, just as progesterone levels are beginning to rise.

Progesterone reaches its peak around day twenty-four or twenty-five; at this point, if fertilization has not occurred, LH shuts down, the corpus luteum withers, and progesterone levels drop sharply. Meanwhile, estrogen levels will have gradually reached their lowest point as well: When both have hit bottom, menstruation occurs.

The Menstrual Cycle

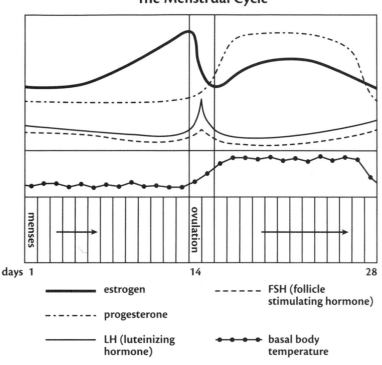

- —————— estrogen
- — - — - — - progesterone
- —————— LH (luteinizing hormone)
- — — — — — FSH (follicle stimulating hormone)
- •—•—•—•—• basal body temperature

Another hormone that fluctuates regularly in our bodies is *testosterone*, one of the androgens produced by the adrenal glands (and also by the ovaries). Testosterone levels in women are seldom more than a tenth of those in most men, except in pregnancy when a woman is carrying a male fetus. Testosterone peaks twice within the monthly cycle, once with ovulation and again with menstruation.

Then there is *oxytocin*, another hormone produced by the pituitary. Oxytocin is generated cyclically and, as previously discussed, in response to certain emotional stimuli. It peaks with ovulation, and as one of its actions is to contract the uterus, it is also elevated immediately before and during menstruation. It enhances fertility in women by increasing movement of the fallopian tubes, and it increases the sperm count in men when given by nasal spray. It spikes with orgasm, and is ten times higher during childbirth than any other time in a woman's life (for more on this fascinating hormone see page 55).

Perhaps the "mother of all hormones" is *dehydroepiandrosterone (DHEA)*, as our bodies can transform it into any other sex hormone. Like testosterone, it is a steroid hormone, made primarily by the adrenals but also by the ovaries. Although DHEA cycles throughout the day, it has no particular correlation to the menstrual cycle. It is thought to be responsible for mediating the ebb and flow of other sex hormones, lending continuity to sexual behavior and communication. DHEA is present in all mammals, but humans are unique in that levels are equal in males and females. This may partially explain the more continuous sexual receptivity of women as compared to that of other mammals.

Physical Changes Throughout the Cycle

◎

Now that the key hormones are in place, let's look at how they affect us at different points in the cycle. Keep in mind that the twenty-eight-day cycle is fairly common but far from standard; cycles may run as short as twenty-one days or longer than forty. Fluctuations in cycle length from month to month are also normal.

Menstruation itself may last as few as three days or as many as seven. Women with longer periods often have a break in the middle when the flow stops before resuming for a day or two. Immediately after menstruation ends, most women have several days with little or no vaginal secretion. The fertility awareness method calls these dry days, which are generally safe from risk of conception—but if you want to make love during this time, you need ample stimulation to lubricate. Depending on how long menstruation lasts and the overall length of the cycle, dry days may be numerous or entirely absent. How so? Take a look at the chart on page 39, which compares the cycles of several different women. Note that regardless of overall

Sample Menstrual Cycles

DAY	DISCHARGE		
	Average/ Long Cycle	Short Cycle	Stress-Affected Cycle
1	menses	menses	menses
2	menses	menses	menses
3	menses	menses	menses
4	menses	spotting	spotting
5	menses	menses	dry
6	spotting	menses	dry
7	dry	spotting-slick	slippery
8	dry	slick	moist
9	dry	stretchy	moist
10	dry	dry	damp
11	dry	dry	dry
12	dry	dry	dry
13	creamy	dry	stretchy
14	creamy	dry	slippery
15	wet-milky	dry	wet
16	slippery	dry	dry
17	stretchy	gummy	dry
18	dry	gummy	dry
19	gummy	dry	pasty
20	dry	slippery	gummy
21	pasty	damp	dry
22	pasty	menses	dry
23	gummy		dry
24	dry		dry
25	dry		dry
26	dry		dry
27	dry		dry
28	damp-spotting		menses
29	slick		
30	menses		

cycle length, ovulation occurs fourteen days before menstruation begins. Barring disease or other abnormal conditions, this time span is biochemically fixed. Variation occurs in the preovulatory phase, where length of menstruation and the number of both dry and preovulatory days may be somewhat unpredictable.

Preovulatory days are generally characterized by a buildup of white, creamy vaginal secretion. Gradually, this is replaced by a clear, slippery, and profuse fertile mucus, which looks something like egg white. Ovulation takes place when fertile mucus reaches peak levels, at which time it has a unique quality known as "spin" (from the German *spinnbarkeit*): If you take a bit of it between your fingers and then pull your fingers apart, it will stretch to form a strand. This mucus has the same alkaline pH as seminal fluid, and the perfect molecular structure for sperm to swim through. It can also keep sperm living in the vagina for up to five days. This is why, when using fertility awareness as a contraceptive method, you must abstain or use protection at the first sign of secretion after your dry days. You never know when this mucus will shift to fertile, and when it does, any sperm in the vaginal canal or cervical crypts (small pockets within the cervical opening) can be kept viable until an egg is released.

Fertile mucus is present for approximately five to seven days, and then it shifts abruptly to a drier, stickier, yellow-white secretion. Nevertheless, a woman is not safe from risk of conception until three and a half of these postovulatory days have passed, allowing time for the more acidic pH of this mucus to kill off any remaining sperm. In a twenty-eight-day cycle, this brings us to about day nineteen or twenty.

The rest of the month is characterized by the same stickier mucus—with one exception. Just before menstruation begins, some women note a secretion that closely resembles fertile mucus. This is actually a mucus plug from the cervix, which has served to protect the uterus from infection. It is shed spontaneously as progesterone levels fall, at which point menstruation is set to begin.

An important aside: It takes time—at least six months of careful observation—to know your cycle well enough to be able to use fertility awareness as a contraceptive method (or to use a barrier method only when at risk of pregnancy). It is easy to get confused in the beginning: Fertile mucus looks very much like arousal lubrication, and infection can also alter the appearance of vaginal and cervical secretions. Allow enough time to get to know what is normal for you so that you can easily distinguish these variations.

Besides changes in secretion, women also experience fluctuations during the cycle in breast size, weight, pelvic sensations, and body temperature. At midcycle, some breast tenderness and enlargement may occur due to water retention, which can lead to a pound or two of weight gain (as estrogen levels fall, these effects diminish). Also noteworthy is the midcycle, ovulatory sensation of *mittelshmerz,* which may range from a subtle twinge to a strong cramping feeling as an egg is released.

Breast and weight changes later in the cycle are partially due to a second peak of estrogen and are further exaggerated by the increasing presence of progesterone. Progesterone is known as a heat-producing hormone, and high levels may cause a noticeable rise in body temperature. In contrast, when levels plunge premenstrually, women typically experience cold hands and feet.

There are other physiological changes that account for the usual premenstrual symptoms. High levels of androgens may cause intestinal cramping or diarrhea; conversely, some women experience constipation in this phase. Androgens also cause expansion and constriction of blood vessels; as levels fluctuate, women may experience headaches, inflammation of varicose veins, or rapid heartbeat.

A common question from women in their mid-thirties is why PMS is getting worse, or if never a problem before, is suddenly noticeable for the first time. As we age, the midcycle estrogen peak soars higher, while the second rise tends to diminish. With less estrogen in the luteal phase, effects of progesterone and the androgens become more exaggerated. Very young women tend to experience similar effects but for a different reason—their bodies are still maturing, so they have less estrogen to modify relatively high testosterone/androgen levels.

During menstruation, progesterone and estrogen are at their lowest levels (although the pituitary gland is primed to release FSH and set the cycle in motion once again). It is interesting that this hormonal low point is literally a fallow phase, a time that allows for rest and rejuvenation both physically and emotionally.

Emotional and Sexual Mood Swings

◎

Perhaps you have already begun to link these physical changes to your own patterns of emotional and sexual response. As menstruation ends and dry days begin, it's no wonder that many women don't feel much like making love. After all, vaginal dryness isn't particularly erotic, and on a purely physical level, the hormonal upswing has just begun. Energetically, though, many women find the preovulatory phase a great time to formulate ideas, make plans, and get busy. As estrogen and testosterone increase, the drive is there to get things done.

Accordingly, ovulation is the high point of the month, a time of peak performance. The skill of manipulating small objects increases dramatically as estrogen levels rise.[1] Women in their fertile phase also experience peak cognitive abilities.[2] The physical effects of fertility—elevated body temperature, fullness and sensitivity of the breasts, the slippery wetness of the vagina as though already aroused—further increase women's feelings of vitality, desirability, and self-confidence. All systems are "Go" when we are fertile: We are physically "in heat," and if our genitals were exposed and visible to potential partners, telltale signs both visual and olfactory would signal biological receptivity.

Women unaware of the cycle of mucus changes often think they are developing an infection during the fertile phase. It's not that the secretion is offensive, but it is profuse and tends, when exposed to air and kept warm (as in underwear), to develop a rather musky odor. One woman graphically described this as a "barnyard smell," sweet and somewhat strong. Women's sense of smell is consistently more acute than men's, but at ovulation it is especially sharp and attuned (in heterosexual women, at least) to the classically male musk odor known in its synthetic form as exaltolide.

Needless to say, this is a great time for lovemaking. As Sharon says, "It's the time I'm always ready. I don't need foreplay because I'm already wet, but the more I have, the more powerful my orgasm." The intensity of orgasm is partially correlated to the estrogen peak, which stimulates circulation in the pelvic area, including the vaginal tissues, which become swollen with blood and warmer than usual. The internal muscles also become more sensitive and responsive. And the testosterone peak at this time further increases assertiveness and self-confidence, as well as sexual thoughts and fantasies.

Emotionally, a majority of women say they feel decidedly amorous while ovulating. As Sara describes it, "For me, there is both passion and tenderness. I really want Tom, but I don't feel tense or rushed about it. I feel ripe and full, with passion everywhere in my body. I feel like playing and taking my time, because I know I'm geared for maximum sensation and incredible orgasm."

Women typically describe the orgasms they have when fertile as "deep in my vagina," "at the core," or "a total body experience." One woman adds, "I feel like my whole body, all of me, is one giant sexual receptor." Another states, "I feel sacred when I'm fertile, like all of me is at its best. I feel integrated and free."

Mary vividly describes both her physical and emotional response as "Sweet...like waves of warm honey flowing through me." Another woman notes, "This is the time of the month when I can really move a tremendous amount of energy through my body. Other times when we make love and I come right away, I feel let down. But when I'm fertile, there's so much energy already that I can build it up, spread it out, and keep doing that until my orgasm is a total thing, it just carries me off completely." "Totality" and "sweetness" are linked to high estrogen levels. Intense desire for sex, pure lust, correlates to the testosterone peak.

This discussion would not be complete without mentioning the pheromones. These olfactory stimulants of desire are released in perspiration and are concentrated in the armpits and genital areas of both men and women, particularly in pubic hair (something to consider as per shaving or depilatory practices). Pheromones are produced by DHEA; they act on the brain through a small cavity inside each of our nostrils, the vomeronasal organ. We can't smell pheromones the way we smell flowers, but we register their chemical messages nonetheless. In women, estrogen causes pheromones to surge midcycle.

In 1986 Winnifred Cutler discovered that male pheromones could serve to regulate female menstrual cycles. With just a bit of pheromone essence (collected from male sweat samples) placed under their nostrils, 70 percent of women with irregular cycles became regular in a matter of months. In a similar vein, in 1971 Martha McClintock demonstrated menstrual synchrony among women sharing quarters in college dorms, due to the effects of their pheromones. Even more intriguing is the finding that in monogamous heterosexual couples, sexual rhythms tend to synchronize, with male testosterone surges matching female estrogen and progesterone surges, largely in response to pheromone exposure.[3]

Hormones and pheromones aside, there is another aspect to heightened desire at midcycle. Particularly in partnerships founded on love, passion may spring from the awareness of our fertility and the knowledge that we have the power to conceive—not necessarily the intent, but the power to recreate ourselves. Listen to what Ellen has to say: "Just knowing I'm fertile gets me completely turned on. This is the time when I most feel the power of creation flowing through me. Once my partner is aware, he intensifies my feelings with his own. We use condoms, and sometimes we 'play the edges' by having long, drawn-out foreplay—there's an element of danger and excitement in being unprotected until we finally get the condom in place. The charge we build up, the intimacy, is really something else!"

For lesbians, synchronous cycling can lead to mutual fertile times, with exponentially increased sexual and emotional potential. Meg says, "Sex when we're fertile is a blast, we are both so wet and open, the desire just flows."

But for some heterosexual couples, the flip side of this passion may be the challenge of using contraception in that it may feel like a betrayal or, at the very least, a bit of a letdown. Especially if a couple has children already and fully understands the potential of this time, or if one wants another child while the other does not, the emotional content of midcycle sex can be rather explosive.

We will look more at contraceptive methods and issues later in this chapter. For now, suffice to say that the fertile time is indeed a power point. Apart from sexual activity, some women plan key business meetings, important family events, holidays, or new ventures to coincide with this phase. From Gina: "I'd been observing my cycles for a long time, four years maybe, when I finally realized I had more energy and did my best work on the upswing from when my period ended on through ovulation. What's even more interesting is that part of me has incorporated the rhythm of my cycle in my day-to-day planning—I don't even have to think about it anymore."

Does this mean that the postovulatory phase is merely a downhill slide? Not entirely, although progesterone (which peaks about ten days after ovulation) and other substances from the adrenals called *aldosterones* do tend to dampen desire. Christiane Northrup describes the luteal phase as "reflective...we turn more inward, preparing to develop or give birth to something that comes from deep within ourselves."[4] Thus women may report less interest in sex in the second part of the cycle.

But several days before menstruation, when progesterone levels decrease and testosterone increases dramatically, many women notice another sexual peak. When asked to characterize it, they say, "hot," "intense," "urgent," "driving," or "very physical." Samantha says, "Right before my period, I feel, I don't know, more masculine in my approach to sex, more aggressive." And from Joan: "I want it fast, hot, physically rough.... I come quickly, explosively...it's great!" Ann observes, "I'm less emotional about sex—really, I just want to get off." Testosterone moves us to pursue, initiate, or dominate, with a focus on genital sex.

There is, by the way, an interesting relationship between testosterone and spatial skills, which increase dramatically under its influence.[5] This may explain women's increased tendency at this time to both envision and enact sexual scenarios.

Mild premenstrual symptoms such as heightened sensitivity of the skin, especially the breasts and nipples, may further increase sexual pleasure. Many women prefer being on top at this time so they can control the depth and angle of penetration, and the rate of clitoral stimulation. Plus, there is more opportunity in this position for being touched and admired. On the other hand, if premenstrual symptoms are severe, any amount of stimulation may be too much until menstruation is under way.

Premenstrual Syndrome

A few words about premenstrual syndrome (PMS): Some experts believe low progesterone levels to be the primary cause. Insufficient progesterone in the monthly cycle may or may not cause premenstrual irritability but definitely links to episodes of breakthrough bleeding several days before menstruation begins (remember, progesterone's job is to maintain the uterine lining). Increasing numbers of women in my practice report these symptoms occasionally, some chronically. Oddly enough, lab tests don't always corroborate clinical symptoms of deficiency. I speculate that even though progesterone levels appear to be within normal range, they are low relative to excessively high levels of synthetic estrogen in our bodies. For example, BGH/BST is used to speed growth and plump up beef and poultry, with residues highly concentrated in eggs, milk, and milk products. An obvious solution is to minimize consumption of these foods or look for grass-fed or free-range alternatives.

We are additionally exposed to high levels of xenoestrogens in our groundwater. These are derived from the manufacture and breakdown of plastics, pesticides, PCBs, and dioxin, and may be stored in our fat cells indefinitely. It is difficult to avoid exposure to the xenoestrogens, which are believed to play a major role in the increasingly early onset of menarche and the rise in breast and prostate cancers. Drinking filtered or bottled water, eating food that has been irrigated with pure water as it is grown, and avoiding fish harvested from polluted waters (especially shellfish) can help us avoid exposure. It is also wise to minimize the use of products containing dioxin, which occurs in the bleaching process used to whiten toilet paper, paper towels, tampons, and other products.[6]

Here are some other recommendations to avoid xenoestrogen exposure:

o Stop using insecticides, pesticides, and chemical lawn-care products. Most insecticides have xenoestrogenic effects.

o Stop eating any product that contains BHA (butylated hydroxyanisole). This is a common food preservative found in processed foods, and it is a xenoestrogen.

o Don't heat any food in the microwave in a plastic bowl or with plastic wrap on it. Softer plastics leach xenoestrogens into food. Use a glass bowl or container, or consider heating food on the stovetop.

o Avoid PCBs (polychlorinated biphenyls) in paints and oils.

o Avoid sunscreen that contains 4-MBC, a xenoestrogen.

o Remove paraben-containing lotion from your routine.[7]

To sum up, addressing signs of progesterone deficiency by pill, cream, or vaginal suppository is not recommended without lab work to determine both progesterone and estrogen levels. Even so, progesterone therapy has been randomly successful at best: Remember that the pituitary gland masterminds ovarian function, thus dosing the body with hormones will not provide any lasting effect. A better solution may be found in acupuncture treatment, which can prompt the pituitary gland to release FSH and LH at the right time each month. The ovaries may then begin producing estrogen and progesterone spontaneously in appropriate amounts.

Premenstrual Dysphoric Disorder

The above holds true for women diagnosed with premenstrual dysphoric disorder (PMDD). Symptoms of PMDD are no different that those of PMS, but they are more extreme. The most concerning include severe depression, panic attacks, out-of-control rages, or thoughts of suicide. If these characterize your premenstrual phase, get the help of a good therapist and/or physician.

An antidepressant may be prescribed for symptoms of PMDD, but all too often, women experiencing a particularly bad round of PMS end up on Prozac. Prozac works by boosting serotonin levels, but it has side effects, not the least of which are severely decreased sex drive and delayed orgasm. It's a fine line: Low serotonin levels increase sex drive and make orgasm easy, but very low levels may lead to aggressive, irrational, or even violent behavior. Serotonin deficiency in animals induces indiscriminate choice of partner and the compulsion for immediate gratification.[8] Serotonin is also decreased by dieting or food restriction (here's a good reason to keep eating premenstrually). It may be possible to treat low serotonin levels nutritionally with the amino acid L-tryptophan. L-tryptophan can be dangerous if taken in excess, but certain foods, such as turkey, have naturally high amounts.

Minor mood changes are easily correlated to hormonal shifts around menstruation. But might there not also be psychological precursors to PMS, or even PMDD? I recall a client who was quite concerned that she might be pregnant—she was two weeks late and had never missed a period, yet two pregnancy tests came back negative. A few days later she reported this dream: She was in her office, feeling under pressure because of a boom in business. Her papers began blowing around everywhere, and then she heard a voice say, "Just let go." Although she skipped that cycle completely, she then resumed her normal rhythm. Admittedly, this example goes beyond mere PMS, but it illustrates psychological conditions that can cause it to become extreme.

This is a theme I have explored at length in my writings on intuition: The function of the premenstrual phase on a psychic level as a time for letting go, relinquishing control, allowing the end of one cycle to make way for the next. This involves reflecting on recent events, dreaming and developing intentions for the next phase, but most of all, surrendering and allowing the death of outmoded views and ways. Consider again the hormonal influences: After progesterone peaks, both it and estrogen plummet, not by gradual decline but in a harrowing fall. Rising testosterone only compounds the intensity of this, spurring us to ruthlessly reexamine hidden aspects of our significant relationships and ourselves. Making way for the next round means getting out of the way psychically, bottoming out, and returning to essence. This is the basis of cyclic renewal.

Depending on how readily or easily this occurs, sex may or may not seem desirable. As Sandra reports, "Once I know my period is going to start—I'm cramping or spotting a little—I like to wait on making love until it really gets going. I feel like keeping to myself until I've turned the corner. It's an energy thing for me." Quite the opposite, Pat reports, "A day or two before my period—wow, look out—I've got only one thing on my mind!"

Even if our premenstrual symptoms are relatively mild and predictable, we all have a terrible time of it now and then. Screaming at our kids, fighting bitterly with our loved ones, breaking or throwing things, crying in public places—these extremes are often the tail end of a very trying month emotionally, or a time of less than optimal health. Poor health and stress definitely disrupt the metabolism and may thus affect hormonal balance. Keeping tabs on ourselves day to day, not overdoing it, getting enough rest and relaxation all help, but sometimes circumstances call for something more. Take a look at the box below for helpful tips on how to cope with PMS.

Ways to Cope with PMS

1. **Evoke your emotions.** Listen to the most sentimental, moving music you can find, the kind that hits the spot, and let yourself cry, yell, rave if you will. We midwives tell new mothers that letting their tears flow will help their milk come down; the same is true of tears and the menstrual flow.

2. **Experience the dark side.** Review the underbelly of the month, all the things that have hurt you, made you blue, or made you feel powerless or furious. Be aware of accumulated tensions in your psyche and your body.

3. **Note spontaneous resolutions.** As you relive the negative events of your last cycle, note any inspirations for doing it differently or better next time, any spontaneous resolutions. This is a great time for saying, "I'm never going to let _____ happen to me again," or, "I'm not going to do _____ anymore!"

4. **Eat.** Studies have shown that as naturally as women gain a few pounds before menstruating, they lose them immediately after. In one such study, the control group struggled not to respond to food cravings. They didn't gain weight, but they didn't lose weight once menstruation was over, either. You need more calories at this time. Many women report cravings for green vegetables, as well as foods high in calcium and protein, which can balance chocolate and sugar splurges that provide only a temporary lift.

(cont'd.)

5. **Exercise.** A full-body, aerobic routine is especially good premenstrually. Aerobic exercise stimulates circulation and elimination, thus counteracting symptoms like backache, bloating, cramping, and fatigue.

6. **Stay warm.** To compensate for circulatory changes, stay cozy. Wear socks, wrap up in a blanket, take a sauna, turn up the heat, and wear loose, nonconstricting clothing (no tight jeans, tight shoes, tight bras, etc.).

7. **Make space for yourself.** Take time off, find ways to defer your responsibilities, or duck out of them completely if they are truly excessive. Clear the decks! And make time to be alone, do the things that make you feel good. In a word, indulge.

8. **Have sex if you want to.** A little sex goes a long way in alleviating premenstrual tension. But be yourself—weepy, passionate, outrageous, outspoken—and make sex work for you. Masturbate, enjoy your body.

9. **Celebrate when your period begins.** Do some sort of letting-go-of-the-old ritual: burn letters, discard objects that symbolize entanglement, make affirmations of new beginnings.

Sex During Menstruation

This brings us to the topic of sex during menstruation, one of our most persistent cultural taboos. Men are still influenced by antiquated beliefs that depict association with menstruating women as a brush with the dark side. Old fears run deep—in biblical times menstruating women were considered unclean, as was anything they touched. Up until a few decades ago, physicians cautioned that sex at this time might lead to infection, advice that has no basis in fact.

Under the laws of Moses, sex was strictly forbidden during, and for a week after, the period. Since a woman's primary function at the time was to produce as many children as possible, it's likely her chances were intensified by avoiding her husband until midcycle when she was fertile, and when his sperm count had had opportunity to increase. Christianity upheld these patriarchal strictures; between the eighth and eleventh centuries, laws denied menstruating women access to church facilities. A Scottish medical text of this period admonished:

> Oh! Menstruating woman, thou'rt a fiend
> From which all of nature should be closely screened.[9]

Many indigenous cultures have also isolated women who are menstruating. Sometimes this has been women's choice; alternatively, cultural taboos removed women from the rest of society. In her fascinating book *Blood, Bread, and Roses: How Menstruation Created the World,* Judy Grahn explains that in Neolithic times, menstruating women were isolated (literally sent up a tree) to protect the rest of the tribe, lest the scent of their blood attract predators.[10] And in other early societies, menstruating women were isolated for being overly powerful and magical: that they could bleed without consequence of illness, debility, or death was utterly confounding and frightening to men. But in matriarchal traditions, the menstrual phase is honored as a time when women unite heavenly and earthly forces: heavenly, in that their bleeding links to lunar cycles; earthly, in that they embody cycles of birth, death, and rebirth found in nature. Before the days of tampons or pads, women often let themselves bleed into the earth, with their blood revered as sacred.

In her wonderful book *Red Flower: Rethinking Menstruation,* Dena Taylor documents a range of women's responses to menstruation. Almost universal is the desire for seclusion: Many spoke of wanting to curl up in bed and relax, sleep by themselves, and avoid going out in public. Some spoke of only wanting to be with women, and how nice it would be to have a special place where they could gather with others who are also menstruating.[11] In many indigenous societies, this was the menstrual hut, which symbolized separation from the ordinary concerns of daily life.

Ernest Hartmann, author of *The Biology of Dreaming*, notes that women dream most between days twenty-five and thirty of the cycle. These dreams are often sexual, aggressive, or even violent, as compared to dreams at ovulation, which tend to be mystical, calming, and more integrative in effect. According to authors Shuttle and Redgrove, dream images during menstruation commonly include talking animals, animals with human heads, violent acts, accidents and delays, and broken objects, whereas ovulating women report dreams of babies, fragile things, jewels, exquisite landscapes, and their mothers.[12] In terms of sexual content, women usually dream about having sex with their partner when ovulating; when menstruating, it's more often sex with a stranger.

Premenstrually, women also dream of death. This makes sense, as it is the lowest point hormonally and the turning point of the cycle as well. When I was still cycling, I was often melancholy at this time of the month: wondering what I would do if one of my children died, or struggling with feelings of despair over difficult situations in my life that I feared would never change. But once I started bleeding, my emotions loosened up and I felt like myself again.

It is important to note that PMS is reportedly more severe when sleep is inadequate. Hartmann asserts that women need more sleep at this time for the natural release of dreaming. Note, however, that tranquilizers and sleeping pills prescribed for PMDD (premenstrual dysphoric disorder) may repress or inhibit dreaming.

Native-American traditions hold the dreams of bleeding women in high esteem. Most tribes believe that a girl's dreams at menarche tell of her mission or direction in life. According to Brooke Medicine Eagle, author and shaman, the most astounding prophetic visions and dreams, including unimaginable events like the coming of the white man, were brought to the people through the "Moon Lodge," women's ritual place of seclusion during menstruation.[13]

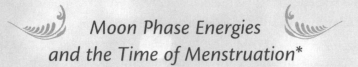

Moon Phase Energies and the Time of Menstruation*

Waxing Moon Menstruation

The waxing moon is a time of growth, of new trends and activities emerging, new beginnings. This is a time to turn inward and tap your own wisdom, a time to learn new skills and make discoveries.

In Native-American cultures, the animal of the waxing moon is the raven, symbolizing exchange of knowledge and flight of the soul. According to the ancient Greeks, the goddess of this phase is Persephone, who walked the underworld.

Full Moon Menstruation

The full moon is outwardly focused: This is a time to bring to bear, to work, and to do. Whereas the waxing moon correlates to daybreak, the full moon is like high noon, a time when things may be revealed. This is a charged and emotionally challenging phase, when the fiercely determined nature of menstruating women is fully evident.

In Native-American cultures, the animal of the full moon is the phoenix, capable of burning to ashes and then rising anew. The full moon goddess of ancient Babylon was Ishtar, also known as the Red Goddess.

Waning Moon Menstruation

The waning moon parallels sunset, when energy subsides and stabilizes. Now is the time to firm up plans, substantiate discoveries, verify knowledge, and let ideas bear fruit.

In Native-American cultures, the animal of this phase is the she-bear who signifies the womb and is therefore pro-

* Adapted from *Dragontime* by Luisa Francia (New York: Ash Tree Publishing, 1988).   (cont'd.)

ductive. In ancient Greek culture, the goddess of this phase is Demeter, who signifies the harvest.

New Moon Menstruation

The new moon is inwardly focused and gives us time for contemplation, reflection, and germination. This is the midnight phase, one of rest and recuperation. Subconscious memories and anxieties rise to the surface; significant events are reviewed.

According to Native-American teachings, the animal of this phase is the toad: wise, slippery, solitary, and untouchable due to her poisonous exterior. The goddess is the Greek Hecate, the crone, the trickster, the reaper.

Women's psychic propensity immediately before and during menstruation is, in my opinion, linked to the effects of the hormone oxytocin. As mentioned earlier, this hormone also peaks during ovulation, another time women note great clarity and insight in their work and dealings with others. And many women report visionary moments in afterglow, yet another time when oxytocin peaks (if only momentarily). Oxytocin is a unique hormone in that it is released not only by physiological prompting but also in response to certain emotional stimuli. For example, oxytocin causes the vagina to lubricate and the nipples to harden not only with physical contact, but also at the thought of making love. Thanks to oxytocin, a woman overwhelmed with passion may have an orgasm the moment she is entered, with very little stimulation otherwise. Similarly, breast-feeding mothers reminded of their baby by the cry of another may experience an oxytocin-based letdown of milk. No wonder oxytocin is called the love hormone!

Oxytocin also increases the potential for deeply meditative theta brainwave states.[14] In pregnancy, when oxytocin is at an all-time high, women speak of intuitively knowing their child before it is born, both its gender and its nature. For menstruating women, what society deems raving madness may actually be visionary awareness, or at the very least, the potential for this.

Thus menstruation affords a cyclic opportunity to explore the Mystery, and perhaps, with the right frame of mind and support, a chance to peer into the future. If you are curious about your dreams at this point in your cycle but generally don't remember them, try keeping paper and pen by the bed, or your cell phone for note taking. Be sure to record your recollections immediately upon awaking, even if it's four in the morning (despite what you may think, you won't remember them later).

Many women report yet another peak of sexual activity several days into the menstrual flow. For some, the first two or three days are unappealing because of general messiness, but as the flow shifts from heavy to moderate, passion picks up. Says Nancy, "Frankly, I like sex best when I'm having my period. I don't have to worry about birth control (I know my cycle well), and I'm in a certain mood—bold and steamy. I'm pre-lubricated too, and you know, I don't mind the blood all over everything; it's erotic to me and my partner." Or, as Jane says, "I feel free, I feel primal, I feel connected to my power. The blood turns me on: It's a symbol of life, the color of passion." And from Ana: "Actually, I think it's the hormones coming back around, picking up again. I know it's not the usual image, but I feel fresh, renewed. I don't think about the past, I think about the future."

Some experts suggest that taboos on intercourse during menstruation may have been due to women's unbridled libido and increased orgasmic capacity, causing inordinate male attention and resulting social disruption.[15] On the other hand, Tantric traditions hold that the most powerful sexual rites require that women be menstruating for the "blending of female red and male white."[16]

Referring to Nancy's statement above, a major area of confusion for many women regards whether or not conception is possible during menstruation. This was one of the questions most often missed by the public on the 1990 nationwide Kinsey Sex Quiz. The correct answer is yes, although rarely does this occur. Our bodies don't menstruate and ovulate simultaneously, but the two can occur back to back. For example, a woman with a twenty-one-day cycle could ovulate as early as day six or seven (remember that the postovulatory phase is usually fourteen days). On day five of her menstrual flow, she might already have pre-fertile mucus that could keep sperm viable until an egg is released a day or two later. Conception before day three is virtually unheard of, particularly when the flow is heavy. Yet fear of pregnancy may prevent women from enjoying the free days that do exist at this time and making the most of them.

This brings us full circle on our hormonal journey, once around a typical cycle. Women suffering from gynecological problems and illnesses have different configurations, though, as do those under the influence of certain contraceptive methods.

Health Problems That Affect the Cycle

◎

Failure to menstruate is called amenorrhea. It may be caused by insufficient body fat, tumors of the hypothalamus or pituitary gland, thyroid disease, diseases affecting the central nervous system, diabetes or other chronic diseases, destruction of the endometrium (uterine lining) by excessive curettage (as used in D&C procedures or abortions), drug or alcohol addiction, adrenal disorders, ovarian cysts, or certain medications. Stress or rigorous athletic training occasionally causes a missed period.

There are other diseases and conditions that don't always cause amenorrhea but strongly affect the cycle. *Endometriosis* is fairly widespread and is a major cause of infertility. In women with this condition, for reasons not entirely understood, some portion of the menses flows up into the fallopian tubes and out the tube ends, and endometrial tissue then embeds or implants either in the tubes or outside on the pelvic organs. These implants continue to go through cyclic changes, but since there is no way for the menses they generate to be shed, they scar over repeatedly until adhesions, or abnormal attachments, begin to form between the pelvic structures. Adhesions may cause the uterus or tubes to twist, may prevent eggs from being released or moved down the tubes, or may lead to the development of ovarian cysts, which ultimately disrupt ovulation.

What causes endometriosis? One explanation is a tightly closed cervix, due to scarring from pelvic infection or traumatic abortion, preventing normal menstrual flow. Other theories include that of *müllerianosis,* which posits that the condition begins in the embryonic phase of life, and *coelomic metaplasia,* which suggests that it results from cell transformation due to irritation. Symptoms of endometriosis include abnormal bleeding and pain—with ovulation, menstruation, penetration/intercourse, or bowel movements. Birth control pills or other medications may prove helpful, but alternative treatments of acupuncture, homeopathy, and herbs often work as well or better. Pregnancy may also effect a cure, since the hormonal changes of childbearing tend to shrink the implants down to nothing.

Ovarian cysts are fairly common, with symptoms similar to endometriosis but with midcycle pain outstanding—a consistent, nagging sensation low in the pelvis, usually on one side only, which may increase with sexual activity. Ovarian cysts, much like breast cysts (as in fibrocystic disease) may be reduced or eliminated with a combination of aerobic exercise, stress reduction, and improved nutrition with all caffeine sources removed from the diet. Acupuncture may help too, although cysts should also be monitored with bimanual exam lest they grow large enough to rupture, which may permanently damage the ovary.

Polycystic ovarian disease, or *Stein-Leventhal syndrome,* is characterized by major hormonal imbalances and amenorrhea. Low FSH, high estrogen, erratic surges of LH, low progesterone, and elevated male hormones virtually eliminate the cycle. In this disease, follicles swell but fail to release eggs, then fill with fluid and become cysts. Cells around the eggs produce testosterone that converts to estrogen, fooling the body into thinking ovulation is about to occur. The pituitary responds by cutting back on FSH and releasing LH, which normally would cause an egg to break free. But this does not happen; instead, the follicle cyst continues to enlarge. At worst, the cyst might rupture and cause internal bleeding. At the same time, high estrogen levels prevent the uterine lining from shedding, so there are no menses, and this buildup of the endometrium increases the risk of uterine cancer.

How might a woman know she has polycystic disease? Often, the cyst (or cysts) will cause pain or discomfort in the pelvic region. Amenorrhea and abnormal growth of facial or body hair (in response to elevated testosterone) are other telltale signs.

Yet another circumstance that drastically alters a woman's cycle is *hysterectomy*. In the vast majority of cases, even if the uterus is diseased, the ovaries are fine and should be left in place so that normal hormonal production may continue. But if all the reproductive organs are removed, immediate menopause ensues. For further information on complete hysterectomy, see Chapter 7.

Endometrial hyperplasia occurs when the normal uterine lining is replaced by an overgrowth of glandular tissue. This is caused by high levels of estrogen unbalanced by progesterone, resulting from anovulatory cycles. The primary symptom is irregular and intermittent bleeding, as some parts of the lining behave as though it were day three, others, day twenty-eight, and so on. Most cases of endometrial hyperplasia resolve spontaneously, although a biopsy is recommended to rule out cell abnormality. This condition should definitely be followed closely to make sure it is abating, as women with history of anovulatory cycles have a higher incidence of uterine cancer. Some physicians prescribe progesterone prophylactically (there are also natural progesterone creams). If bleeding becomes chronic, a D&C may help by giving the uterus a fresh start.

Uterine fibroids may also cause bleeding apart from menstruation, making it difficult to track the cycle. Bleeding from fibroids is often correlated to sexual activity. Although fibroids are usually benign, an ultrasound to determine their exact size and location is a good idea, particularly if bleeding is excessive. Pregnancy tends to increase the size of fibroids, whereas menopause reduces them. If fibroids grow so large as to impinge uncomfortably on other pelvic organs (one of the largest documented weighed in at one hundred pounds), surgical removal by myomectomy is an option. Hysterectomy is rarely necessary, and many women with fibroids prefer to wait and see. Dr. Christiane Northrup recommends a three-month trial of a high-fiber, whole-foods diet, eliminating all refined sugar and flour and all dairy products or meats adulterated by hormones. This diet is also recommended for women with endometriosis.[17]

Beyond these conditions, other factors can affect the cycle. Artificial lighting may disrupt lunar regulation of the cycle, particularly if there is a streetlight outside the bedroom window. Opaque blinds can be used to regulate the amount of light in the room; they should be fully open at the full moon and closed completely at the new moon.

And then there is the busy pace of life, which occasionally turns grueling and causes us to lose touch with our personal rhythms, those times during the day when we naturally seek food, rest, or stimulation. Some people are morning types, some more nocturnal. Frequently, our personal rhythms are at odds with our social routine; we may not, for example, feel like eating at traditional meal times.

Learning to follow our rhythms is important. Many women in my practice say they would do anything for time alone, a day off once in a while to do exactly as they please. My advice is to take the time before it is too late! In terms of optimal health, following our subtle instincts makes all the difference: seeing that we have exactly what we want to eat, finding privacy for a few moments when we most need it, or taking a second or two to breathe deeply.

Overindulgence in junk food, sugar, coffee, or alcohol can obscure our rhythms and instincts by stressing and debilitating our bodies, causing us to lose needed vitamins and minerals. When we are less than healthy, our emotional reactions become extreme, and our abilities to handle life's challenges become impaired. Mood elevators like Prozac interfere with our biorhythms and, if overused, can exacerbate the very emotional problems they are intended to alleviate.

It is unfortunate that most of us know little of the healing properties of tonic and medicinal herbs, but this is relatively easy to remedy. Herbs are allies for health and harmony; when we use them wisely, desires for harmful substances or less-than-healthful foods may begin to fall away. There are many fine beginning texts on herbology; explore them online or at your local bookstore or library.

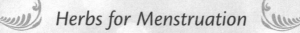

Herbs for Menstruation

With all herbs, source and processing make all the difference. Familiarize yourself with any herb farms in your area, and seek out distributors who carry organic products. Good tinctures are dated for reference and generally appear clear, not muddy.

Basil (*Ocimum bascilicum*), particularly the fresh leaf, stimulates bleeding, invigorates, and lifts feelings of depression. A favorite way to take basil is in pesto; served with pasta it is especially good at the onset of menstruation as the carbohydrates provide calories and warmth.

Catnip (*Nepeta cataria*) is pain killing, cramp easing, soothing, and calming. It calms digestive disturbances caused by aldosterones (and is thus renowned for its ability to ease colic in newborns). Take as a tea or tincture.

(cont'd.)

Ginger (*Zingiber officinale*) stimulates circulation, warms and balances the body, and also helps dispel gastrointestinal upsets. Take fresh in food or tea, or dried in capsules.

Life root (*Senecio aureus*) is best taken by tincture: Five to ten drops daily help to regulate the cycle and ease PMS. It may also relieve severe cramps, uterine or intestinal. Herbal lore teaches that life root blossoms were found carefully placed on the oldest grave known.[18] It is especially effective if taken long-term.

Motherwort (*Leonurus cardiaca*) is most effective taken by tincture: Take ten drops to relax, fifteen drops to ease menstrual pain. Motherwort is also used for hot flashes during menopause and to ease labor pains.

Nettle (*Urtica dioica*) helps rid the body of excess water while strengthening the kidneys and adrenals. It also provides vitamin K, carotene, protein, and key minerals for menstruation, such as calcium and iron. It is especially useful for excessive bleeding.

Raspberry (*Rubus species*) is said to represent women's passion and life force. Raspberry tea eases PMS and tones the uterus; it is mood elevating and elicits, according to Luisa Francia, "passionate menstruation." It is the beverage of choice for women during pregnancy and postpartum.

Rosemary (*Rosmarinus officinalis*), in either the oil or leaf form, is strengthening and stabilizing to the body. It stimulates bleeding and helps keep energy high and consistent during menstruation.

The Effects of Contraceptive Methods

◎

No discussion of contraception would be complete without mention of safe sex as protection from hepatitis B and C, HIV, and other sexually transmitted infections. Although condoms and latex dams are simple enough in concept, some women have difficulty insisting on their use. This is dangerous, as the incidence of AIDS has risen dramatically among heterosexual women.

The need to take last-minute precautions changes sexual dynamics, particularly those of foreplay. Ideally, a couple should discuss safe sex in advance, but often the subject arises concurrently with passion. A number of my clients report being surprised at how bringing up safe sex sets them on equal footing with their male partners: Conventional roles of man as aggressive and woman as passive shift dramatically. Foreplay then becomes playful, and acts of securing the condom or placing the dam can be humorously erotic.

The Female Condom

Although barrier methods are surveyed later in this section, the female condom bears mention here. This device consists of a sheath of latex with one open and one closed end, each encircled by a rubber ring. The smaller ring (at the closed end) is inserted and placed over the cervix; the larger ring remains outside the body, resting over the labia. The newest version is called the FC2: Made of nitrile, it is softer than the original polyurethane version. Clinical studies in the United States and Japan show that it is 95 to 98 percent effective when used correctly and consistently. Some women report discomfort during intercourse, presumably from the outer ring rubbing against the labia or clitoris—still, the female condom gives a woman the prerogative.

The Pill, the Patch, the Vaginal Ring, and Injectable Contraceptives

Regarding the more popular contraceptives, we will start with hormonal methods: the Pill, the Patch, the Ring, and injectables. Put bluntly, these completely obliterate the cyclical pattern of emotional and sexual response presented earlier in this chapter. Most formulas combine estrogen and progestin to create a state of pseudo-pregnancy, with hormone levels high enough to trick the body into believing it has already conceived so that ovulation will not occur. Excess estrogen may cause weight gain, breast tenderness, nausea, headaches, fatigue, and more serious health problems; excess progesterone has side effects as well (see the box below).

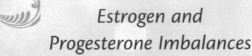

Estrogen and Progesterone Imbalances

Please be aware that isolated symptoms may not have significance, whereas a combination of symptoms is more indicative of imbalance.

Signs of Estrogen Excess

- nausea and vomiting
- dizziness
- edema
- leg cramps
- increase in breast size
- chloasma (brown pigmentation on face)
- changes in eyesight
- hypertension
- certain headaches (vascular)

Signs of Estrogen Deficiency

- early spotting (days one to fourteen)

(cont'd.)

o reduced menstrual flow

o nervousness

o painful intercourse due to vaginal changes

Signs of Progesterone Excess

o increased appetite

o tiredness

o depression, mood changes

o breast tenderness

o vaginal yeast infection

o oily skin and scalp

o hirsutism (excess body hair)

Signs of Progesterone Deficiency

o late spotting and breakthrough bleeding (days fifteen to twenty-one)

o heavy menstrual flow, with clots

o decreased breast size

You may be thinking, "Wait a minute...apart from the high hormone levels created by the Pill, aren't the combination formulas designed to give women something of a cycle?" Yes, but not a natural one: These formulas are designed merely to alternate negative impacts of the hormones involved. If you are on the Pill and are wondering which type you have, here is a guide:

o *Monophasic (one-phase) pills* contain the same amount of estrogen and progestin. Alesse, Loestrin, Ortho-Cyclen are a few examples.

o *Biphasic (two-phase) pills* change the level of estrogen and progestin once each cycle. Examples are Kariva and Mircette.

o *Triphasic (three-phase) pills* contain three different doses
   of hormones, changing every seven days during the first
   three weeks (this was the original formula). Examples are
   Cyclessa, Ortho Tri-Cyclen, Nortel, Enpresse, and Ortho-
   Novum.

o *Quadraphasic (four-phase) pills* change hormone levels four
   times per cycle. Natazia is the only such product in the U.S.
   market.

o *Progestin-only pills,* or *mini-Pills,* are usually suggested for
   nursing mothers, or for women with pre-existing risks or
   other conditions that prevent them from taking estrogen.
   They must be taken with strict regularity (same exact same
   time every day) to prevent ovulation, but they also work by
   thickening the cervical mucus so the sperm cannot reach the
   egg, and by changing the lining of the uterus so that implantation of a fertilized egg is unlikely to occur.

This brings us to the Yaz/Yasmin/Ocella scandal. These all include drospirenone, a form of progesterone now linked to heart attack, stroke, deep vein thrombosis (DVT), cerebral venous sinus
thrombosis (CVT), and death (numerous lawsuits are pending).
Women also report missing periods for months on end. A marketing ploy used by Bayer to encourage use of these products was relief
from PMDD, which, even if true, hardly justifies the risks! If you are
taking these Pills, find an alternative at once.

And what about the formulas that suspend menstruation for
months at a time, like Seasonale and Seasonique, or Lybrel, which
stops it indefinitely? Consider the more serious side effects of the
Pill in general, such as stroke, heart attack, liver damage, blood clots
and thromboses, and how these might be exacerbated with little or
no break from exposure. Implants such as Nexplanon (which offers
protection for three years) also fall into this category, as does Depo-
Provera, an injectable that offers protection for three months.

In checking the side effects of Lybrel, I was shocked to find that
the one clinical trial in North America involved only 2,134 subjects,

more than half of which (58.6 percent) discontinued use during the one-year span. Evaluations were for contraceptive effectiveness and relief from menstruation (nothing on other health impacts), with just a 60 percent success rate of amenorrhea. The remaining 40 percent experienced random breakthrough bleeding—hardly the effect promised by the advertising![19]

Building on the theme of little-disclosed side effects: The vaginal ring (otherwise known as the Ring, or NuvaRing) may be associated with an increased risk for vaginal cancer, as chronic irritation of the vagina, experienced by some users, predisposes to this condition.[20] And Depo-Provera is linked to bone density loss that may or may not be reversible: just another example of "market first, warn later."

Whatever the formula—the Pill, the patch, the vaginal ring, or injectables—all maintain a hormonal pattern foreign to a woman's own. Gone are the natural peaks of estrogen, oxytocin, and testosterone. Gone are the creativity and passion of ovulation, the intense, red-hot desire immediately before or during menstruation. Gone too are the psychological benefits of phasing through the cycle, of cyclic completion and renewal. When it comes to the "period" experienced with the Pill, this is merely breakthrough bleeding when hormone levels drop temporarily, as only ovulation can trigger the buildup and subsequent release of the uterine lining that is menstruation.

When my clients speak of a desire to get off these methods, they often cite the primary reason as wanting to be more in touch with their bodies. The more we talk, the more it becomes clear that what they really miss is being in touch with themselves, nuances of feeling they once enjoyed, their own unique mind-body blend. It's disturbing to consider the extent to which dosing women with artificial hormones can modify personality and sexual response, but such is clearly the case.

As for the latter, we have ample clinical confirmation of loss of libido in women using hormonal contraception. Psychobiologist

Rosemarie Krug (Department of Clinical Neuroendocrinology at the Medical University of Lubeck) studied women's responses to erotic imagery, comparing those on the Pill to those who were not. Three times a month—at ovulation, premenstrually, and with menstruation—participants were shown a series of rapid images of naked men, babies, and women combing their hair, and were asked to categorize their response as sexual, maternal, or body related. Women at ovulation were much quicker to spot the babies and naked men and to read sexual connotations into hair-care images than were women on the Pill, whose sexual responses were at low levels throughout the month, never reaching the intensity of normally cycling women. Krug concluded that the Pill negatively affects libido by lowering testosterone levels and obliterating natural hormonal peaks at ovulation.[21]

Yet another study explored the effects of male pheromones on women using the Pill with those who were not. Male participants were asked to wear a T-shirt for several days without showering or using deodorants or cologne; they also could not smoke or eat spicy foods. The T-shirts were then put into boxes for the women to smell and rate according to appeal. Women not on the Pill were attracted by the scent of men with immune systems unlike, and therefore complementary, to their own, which researchers concluded would naturally benefit their offspring. But women on the Pill chose men with immune systems almost identical to their own. Researchers concluded that women on the Pill behaved as though they were pregnant, choosing men more like kin for the sake of protection, rather than men suitable for mating.[22]

I find the implications of this study to be most significant. These effects of the Pill may be less an issue for the woman already in a relationship, but for the woman still looking for Mr. Right, it's disturbing to think that the Pill or other hormonal methods could prevent her from recognizing him at a crucial biological level.

Hormonal contraception may be therapeutic for certain gynecological problems such as endometriosis or pathologically painful menstruation, but we must remember that relief obtained in these cases merely masks underlying causes. Again, acupuncture (along with dietary changes) may effectively reeducate the system to a more-balanced hormonal state.

Herbal Sources of Estrogen and Progesterone

Please remember that fresh, organic herbs and herb products are best, and that tincture form generally offers the greatest potency.

Herbs That Stimulate Estrogen Production

o blue cohosh

o black cohosh

o basil

o sage

o black currant

o licorice

o raspberry leaf

Herbs That Stimulate Progesterone Production

o sarsaparilla

o wild yam root

o chaste tree (vitex)

Acupuncture may also be useful for women coming off hormones. It is not uncommon for women to miss a period or two when they first discontinue, as the body has forgotten its rhythm and needs to get back on track. If the rhythm is lost for six months or more, acupuncture and herbs can stimulate pituitary secretion of LH and FSH, with subsequent ovarian response. This treatment is definitely preferable to the use of pharmaceuticals. Problems with delayed cyclical function are much more common after the age of thirty—ironically, a time when women often quit contraception to get pregnant. Many women report herbal tinctures of Vitex and cotton-root bark to be helpful in rebalancing the hormonal system.

The IUD

In the United States we have two brands of IUD: the ParaGard (a copper device) and the Mirena (progestogen-releasing). The latter obviously has side effects similar to the mini-pill, while the former does not directly alter hormonal balance. But why do so many women using copper IUDs report heavier and more painful periods than ever before? The official explanation is that these problems are merely mechanical, a result of low-grade irritation sufficient to prevent pregnancy but with side effects of cramping and increased bleeding. The truth is that the copper IUD does not prevent conception but works by preventing implantation. Thus the heavy periods associated with this device may actually be spontaneous miscarriages.

The hormonal effects of this scenario, though indirect, may be quite drastic. If conception does occur, dramatic elevations in estrogen and progesterone levels follow. I had an IUD myself many years ago, and once I pieced this realization together, I couldn't wait to get it out. The idea of miscarrying repeatedly as a method of contraception was both physically and spiritually repugnant to me.

I know that some women consider the IUD a godsend. However, the risks are far from minor: With both types, uterine scarring (from chronic irritation) can lead to infertility, tubal pregnancy or tubal rupture, and, rarely, uterine perforation.

Tubal Ligation

The nearly foolproof method of tubal ligation, long touted as having virtually no side effects, merits closer investigation. Studies have shown a correlation with menstrual cycle disruption, and in rare cases, early menopause. Progesterone levels are known to decrease for six months to a year after the procedure, contributing to severe PMS. Sometimes, levels never return to normal.[23] Still, this is the right choice for some women.

The Diaphragm and the Cervical Cap

What about the barrier methods? Clearly, these have no physiological effect on a woman's cycle. But the minor inconveniences are considerable, including chemical irritation from spermicide, lack of spontaneity, messiness, and reduced sensation.

My extensive experience with the British cervical cap (I ran an FDA-approved study from 1982 to 1986) led me to favor it over other barrier methods. Sadly, it is no longer being manufactured, probably because hormonal methods have become so popular. Compared to the diaphragm, it used very little spermicide, with no additional applications required for repeated intercourse. It could be left in place for several days and was small enough to be virtually undetectable. The American version, or FemCap, is, in my experience, clumsy in design and ill fitting: FDA statistics show only 77 percent effectiveness, which is hardly satisfactory.

But the diaphragm has its problems. A little-known fact is that although it feels snug when first placed, the vagina expands so much with arousal that even an oversized fit will move and slide around freely during intercourse, readily admitting seminal fluid. Thus the spermicide inside becomes so diluted that more must be added before having sex again, in an attempt to catch the sperm before they get over the rim. Having personally used a diaphragm for fourteen years, I know well the frustrations of nagging discomfort and disrupted spontaneity. There were many occasions when I was tempted to leave the diaphragm in the drawer, or just toss it in the trash.

Eventually I realized that much of my resistance was due to reduced levels of sensation while making love. Around this time, news of the G-spot hit the press, and suddenly it all made sense. By virtue of its design, the front rim of the diaphragm must displace the G-spot in order to lodge behind the pubic bone. No wonder I couldn't feel much! Once I learned fertility awareness and could safely use a diaphragm only when necessary, my suspicions were confirmed. Before using the cervical cap, I switched to the smallest sized diaphragm (65), which my cervical placement made secure. The problem was solved, as the rim cleared my G-spot with room to spare. If you'd like to explore alternative diaphragm sizing, look for a health-care provider experienced in this.

Some women prefer to alternate diaphragm and condom use, reporting it feels good to share the responsibility with their partner. A comment from Suzanne:

> My partner and I had run the gamut in birth control, and we ended up with barrier methods for safety's sake. But it didn't feel right to me to always be the one who had to remember, to take charge. It's nice when my partner takes his turn with a condom: I can just sit back and relax, and I like the feeling of my body being completely natural. It helps me enjoy sex more.

As mentioned earlier, some women use fertility awareness as birth control and simply abstain during the ovulatory phase. This may cause considerable frustration, though, as intense desire when fertile must consistently be ignored or expressed in ways other than penetration.

Hormonal Changes by Decade

◎

Thus far, we've explored the sexual mood swings of the monthly cycle in somewhat generic terms. However, the hormonal balances we typically run in our twenties are quite different from those in our thirties or forties—each decade has its sexual flavor. Later chapters will explore the evolution of our sexuality in the context of maturation. For now, here is an overview of the hormonal underpinnings of these changes.

The Twenties

Women are generally more physiologically stable in their twenties than in their teens. Testosterone and estrogen surges have leveled off somewhat, although estrogen levels remain high. At this age, many women tend to feel more sexually receptive than assertive and may be attracted to strong and dominating partners more often than they care to admit. Social factors figure here, in that young women in the prime of their reproductive capacity need care and protection in order to raise their young. It is unfortunate that in our culture, this need is not mediated by the love and support of female family members and peers, which might allow a young woman to more selectively choose her mate.

High levels of estrogen also move women at this age to seek intimacy, which can be difficult to find with men their own age, who are strongly testosterone-driven and thus more inclined to sexual conquest than genuine closeness. But women need intimacy: not only for emotional reasons but also for biological ones—touching, kissing, and caressing prompt the release of oxytocin, which triggers a mutual bonding response. Thus women in their twenties long more for passionate, ecstatic touch rather than raw sex, precisely for the bonding opportunity it affords.

PMS can be a problem at this age if a woman is less than conscious of its effects, particularly if she is living with a partner who must deal with these effects too.

The Thirties

Most women in their thirties begin to come into their sexual power. At the same time, it is the phase of life most noted for overwork, one when the average woman feels she runs all day and never quite catches up. Chronic stress causes DHEA levels to drop, which can lead to decreased levels of testosterone, less pheromone production, reduced sex drive, and less orgasmic capacity. Stress may also precipitate some wicked PMS, which may already be a problem as less estrogen is being produced in the luteal phase to buffer the effects of progesterone and the androgens.

But if stress can be managed or set aside, testosterone levels continue to rise. This can boost a woman's confidence, leading her to worldly success and greater sexual assertiveness than ever before. Orgasm is very important to women in their thirties, as they are now more active than receptive, more sure of their needs, and more intent on satisfaction.

The Forties

For many women, there comes a time in their early forties when PMS takes on new character, apart from stress. As we approach menopause, occasional anovulatory cycles cause our hormones to surge in order to force ovulation to continue. This results in much higher levels of estrogen and progesterone than usual, causing extreme emotional heights and depths as levels drop before menstruation.

Testosterone levels also continue to increase, leading women to be more sexually experimental and aggressive than ever before. Women reach their sexual peak sometime in their forties, much as men do in their late teens/early twenties. This discrepancy may prompt some heterosexual women to seek younger partners; others find that men their own age complement their sexual needs perfectly. (Men in their forties experience a decline in testosterone that unmasks estrogen, leading them to be more touch oriented, sensitive, and receptive than when they were younger.)

The Fifties

The average age of menopause is fifty-two, but women may enter menopause much earlier, even in their late thirties. Major shifts in the cycle occur as menopause approaches, with hormone levels fluctuating daily, much as in adolescence. Missed periods, longer-than-usual periods, and scant, irregular bleeding are all considered normal at this time. As women begin to leave the monthly cycle behind, they experience dramatic mood swings and changing sexual desires (again, much as in adolescence).

The Sixties, Seventies, and Beyond

Women in their sixties and beyond enjoy a liberated sexuality based on postmenopausal stability combined with a continued rise in testosterone. They often report thinking less about sex but loving it more than ever once they are engaged—in other words, they feel less compulsion but more satisfaction.

In order to maintain this experience, they must be physically active, aware of their nutritional needs, and adequately rested. Health maintenance is more work than before, but the benefits are great as emotional and psychological stability lend a comfort and confidence with sex only dreamed of in earlier decades.

◎　◎　◎

In the next chapter, we will look specifically at sex in the childbearing cycle, including the fertility dance leading to conception. Particularly if a woman knows her cycle and recognizes her fertility signals, she will be likely to experience conception as it occurs. We will also consider how out-of-sync desires for conception between partners can affect the tone, ease, and frequency of sexual sharing in relationship.

CHAPTER 4

The Sexuality of Pregnancy and Birth

Being aware of your monthly cycle may lead you to notice biological urges for conception. These desires may emerge only in mid-cycle dreams, or you may find yourself fantasizing about babies and birth with increasing frequency. Sometimes, when the desire for a baby has built up over a period of time, women report startling feelings during lovemaking that conception is imminent, regardless of contraceptive precautions. Some report visions of waiting spirits, or images of their infant or toddler to be. As one woman relayed:

> We were in the midst of lovemaking overwhelming from the moment it began, so very powerful, when suddenly I saw this picture in my mind of a blonde, curly-haired little boy and I knew that I could conceive that child, that it wanted to come to me. I tried to tell my partner about it later, but he wasn't ready to hear it—he thought I was fabricating it, I guess. But I never will forget the intensity, the clarity and ultra-real quality of that moment. From then on, I knew we were destined to have a child together and it was only a matter of time.

No one can really say what brings on such revelations, but they clearly go beyond the physical realm. I think couples deeply in love build up so much intensity in their relationship that it eventually overflows and begins to take form, one way or another. Women speak of this fecund state in somewhat mystical terms. Joanne recalls, "I felt like the veil between worlds, this and another place of souls, began to fall away. Soon, all we had to do was touch, and the awareness of that other place, new life just waiting, was all around us."

Looking back, I clearly recall the exact moment when each of my three children was conceived. Even now, I am surprised by how vivid the memories are, every detail of environment and mood crystal clear, my sensory awareness at its peak. Each time, just moments after orgasm, there was a moment of truth and realization, extraordinary and profound that left me sure and shaking with the knowledge that I was pregnant. There was no turning back: I was forever changed!

My experience is somewhat at odds with the notion of "planned pregnancy," which paints conception as a predictable and controllable occurrence. According to my midwifery clientele, conception happens less by deliberation than by surrender, at least most of the time. Women commonly report, "Well, this wasn't exactly what we planned—it happened a bit sooner (or later) than we expected, but we were open to it, and we're happy."

For others, it's not so easy. Couples with a history of infertility are often so burdened with anxiety and frustration that lovemaking becomes a chore. When they do conceive, it may take them a while to relax into the pregnancy. Women with a history of traumatic abortions may also have difficulty conceiving and accepting conception once it occurs, particularly if they have not come to terms with previous losses. The same may be true of women who have endured repeated miscarriage, at least until the crucial window of potential repeat has passed (see Chapter 9 for suggestions on healing).

Sometimes a woman must face the fact that she stands alone in her desire to conceive. Perhaps she and her partner can't agree on when she should get pregnant, or her partner is having second thoughts about parenthood in general. Frankly, I think we health providers have been remiss in helping women realistically address their biological clock issues. I've had far too many clients in their late thirties or early forties speak wistfully of having children one day when their mate is finally ready or their life is finally in perfect order, only to become severely traumatized when infertility forces them to realize that it's too late (yes, there are alternatives of surrogacy or in vitro fertilization—but these are last resorts for most women and may be financially out of the question).

This confusion regarding readiness for parenthood is endemic to a society that provides little social or financial support for pregnant women or young families. It also reveals our inculcated quest for perfection, enacted in the endless struggle for material prosperity as prerequisite to happiness. But Mother Nature has other designs. She did not intend us to wait to have children until we've mastered life, or we would have them in our fifties and sixties. Parenting itself is a vehicle for personal growth; it teaches us to love unconditionally, to accept small strides over time, and to make the most of the way things are, rather than what we think they should be. These are important lessons in human maturation, otherwise difficult to come by. But women today who find themselves wanting children are often beset with doubts, which are magnified by the "rational" reservations of others. This is more than unfortunate. The reproductive impulse is natural, creative, and a gift to cycling women: It is friend, not foe. We must reframe and reclaim the inherent power of our ability to conceive!

When conception occurs, a complex series of hormonal, physical, and psychological changes begin to take place. These changes profoundly affect a woman's emotional stability and sense of self. Especially at first, pregnancy can make a woman feel like her life has been turned on end. But this is normal; it is part of the process.

Pregnancy is comprised of three trimesters, each lasting approximately thirteen weeks. Each of these trimesters has its challenges and joys, which begin to make sense when the process is viewed as a whole.

The First Trimester

◎

Even though a woman may not appear to be pregnant in the first trimester, dramatic changes are taking place in her body. When conception occurs, progesterone and estrogen levels do not drop as in the monthly cycle but rise to several times the normal amounts. This causes the thyroid gland to enlarge, raising the metabolic rate in order to provide extra energy for fetal development and the other physiological demands of pregnancy. Blood vessels dilate to allow for increased blood volume. The adrenals produce additional aldosterone to counter the sodium loss that would otherwise occur with increased estrogen and progesterone. The latter may explain why a woman may feel less sexual than usual at the beginning of pregnancy, at least for the first few weeks.

But this is not the only reason her desire may be waning. Morning sickness, which occurs as the body adjusts to elevated hormone levels, is hardly conducive to cuddling and carrying on. In fact, a woman may feel exceedingly vulnerable at this stage and may need lots of nurturing. Simple acts of kindness, like being brought toast first thing in the morning, mean more than comfort alone; they are a measure of her partner's commitment, and as such can lead to increased intimacy once nausea is overcome. If she is not partnered, she should make it a point to treat herself exceptionally well.

Other physical changes affect the breasts, particularly the nipples, which become hypersensitive to touch. As Alicia reports: "My breasts are rather small and I'm not that confident about them, but when I'm pregnant, they become a focus in our lovemaking." Cheryl sums it up succinctly: "My partner and I have never gotten more pleasure from my breasts than when I was pregnant."

Another inconvenience of early pregnancy is frequent urination, due to uterine enlargement and pressure on the bladder. However, increased circulation in pelvic tissues as a means for uterine growth can also lead to pelvic engorgement, similar to that in premenstrual or ovulatory phases of the cycle. This can cause a woman to desire deep and forceful penetration, at the same time worrying that this may not be safe. There has been much debate on this subject over the years; notions that intercourse and orgasm have deleterious effects on mother and baby have come and gone. For a while, physicians advised that orgasm be strictly avoided, as the resulting uterine activity might cause oxygen deprivation for the baby. Although it is true that orgasm causes uterine contractions, they are too minor to have any serious effect on placental circulation. Additionally, increases in heart rate and respirations compensate for any adverse effects.

There have also been moralistic admonitions against "exposing the fetus to an atmosphere of carnal desire." Let's hope that one is behind us! Some studies link intercourse in the last trimester to uterine infection, but findings are inconclusive due to variables of stress level, dietary habits, and preexisting health conditions.

On the other hand, if there is a history of miscarriage or episodes of bleeding in the current pregnancy, sexual activity should probably be curtailed, at least for the first trimester. It is important to remember, though, that 25 percent of women have bleeding in early pregnancy, but only 8 to 13 percent miscarry. Particularly if bleeding coincides with the time of the month menstruation would ordinarily occur, there is less cause for concern. In this case, it seems that the body maintains its old rhythm for a while until new hormonal levels are fully established.

If there is a history of premature labor, sexual activity may be forbidden later in pregnancy, depending on whether the cervix shows any signs of premature softening or opening. Sometimes a woman must stay in bed for a while until her baby is ready to be born, with intercourse and orgasm strictly taboo.

Barring these exceptions, sex brings physiological benefits of increased pelvic circulation, release of tension, and internal muscle toning particularly helpful in preparation for birth. There are immense psychological benefits too, which help mediate the scope and speed of emotional transformation. Many couples describe their sexual encounters in pregnancy as re-bonding experiences, akin to those in the initial phase of their relationship. No wonder, for both partners are assuming new roles and discovering certain aspects of each other heretofore unknown. For heterosexual couples, there is the extra boost of not having to think about birth control.

A woman's level of desire in the first trimester may also be related to the sex of her child. At about six to eight weeks, when the brain is developing, male fetuses generate large amounts of testosterone, the level of which is four times that in infancy and childhood.[1] This undoubtedly has some effect on the mother, quite possibly increasing her libido. By the same token, a mother's ability to recognize the sex of her unborn child may have a hormonal basis, since surges of testosterone continue to occur in males at regular intervals during gestation, which are, of course, absent in female fetuses.

Precisely how early pregnancy influences a woman's sexuality further depends on her personality, her self-esteem, her desire for the baby, the stability of her primary relationship(s), and various other psychosocial factors. Often, women in our culture feel somewhat frightened upon confirmation of pregnancy: excited but apprehensive nonetheless. This is a normal reaction, considering that most of us know little or nothing about childbearing until pregnant, have never witnessed a birth, and may never have cared for a baby. Despite the thrill of being pregnant, many women feel anxiety about joining the ranks of our least supported social group: mothers. Newly pregnant women soon learn that society considers motherhood a personal venture that must somehow be done "on the side," squeezed onto an already loaded palette of responsibilities. Thus it is never too early to begin establishing a support system, whether by getting together with other expectant mothers or by forging new alliances with female relatives.

Women's reactions to specific stages of childbearing also vary according to personality type. A physically oriented woman, for example, may find the natural softening of her body and loss of emotional control caused by hormone swings at the onset of pregnancy to be excruciating. She may feel that her body doesn't "work" anymore; no longer can she make her way by physical intent alone. Naturally, this will affect her sexual self-image. For her, the key to adjustment is to express her feelings while learning more about the unique capabilities of her changing body.

Emotionally oriented women are quite the opposite, glorying in the heightened sensitivities of pregnancy. They may enjoy sex more than ever, as long as there are no major upheavals in the relationship. Increased needs for food and exercise may go unnoticed, though, resulting in decreased physical energy and emotional instability, which ultimately affects sexual enjoyment. Emotionally based women must learn to focus on messages from their bodies. They also need concrete, factual information on nutrition and the physiology of pregnancy to offset some tendency toward fanaticism.

Mentally oriented women, with a penchant for control and having everything in place, may make their adaptation by the book and yet feel disoriented by surges of emotion and extreme mental states beyond their experience. They must find a way to explore their feelings, connecting mind and body through dance, movement, massage, or whatever serves to facilitate spontaneity and discovery of the inner voice. This can add an entirely new dimension to their sexual experience.

An oft-underrated aspect of pregnancy is the sweeping effect of elevated hormones on the psyche. Or perhaps we get only the downside, the negative view that paints expectant mothers as borderline crazies: forgetful, hopelessly moody, and foolishly preoccupied. But listen to what pregnant women themselves tell us about their psychological state: "I've never felt better in my life," or, "I feel fulfilled, like I'm really myself at last." Consider how well nonpregnant women feel at the monthly estrogen peak—confident, powerful, creative, physically alert, and strong—and juxtapose this to pregnancy, when estrogen levels soar. Elevated oxytocin and DHEA levels also contribute to a heightened state of being.

The Second Trimester

◎

The midpoint of pregnancy is a time of stability. The essential hormonal and mechanical adjustments have taken place and now begin to blend with the mother's own efforts to eat, exercise, and rest responsively. Women love this phase; they feel wonderful and look radiant. Around twenty weeks, most mothers feel the baby move for the first time, an event known as *quickening*. This is an interesting term, connoting awakening and heightened awareness. Some women say they can sense the baby's personality by how it moves; that they learn its nature by its rhythms of activity and rest. Most women quite naturally incorporate feelings for the baby into lovemaking, as the dyad becomes a triad. Women in the second trimester have exceptional powers of perception, concentration, and recuperation, all of which enhance sexual expression. Greater physical equilibrium also serves to boost libido.

Alice, mother of three, puts it this way:

With each of my pregnancies, I became familiar with my baby a little sooner. The first time, I could barely believe I had a baby in me at all; it was so overwhelming. Then, I remember an incident with my second: I had the flu and was quite sick, and after a rather violent episode of vomiting I said out loud, "Oh, I hope she's all right." Yes, I had a girl! With the last, though, I felt I knew him right from the start. I would tell people that he was very active but sweet, and they'd look at me indulgently. It's easy to see now that I was right.

And what about sex with this awareness? Alice continues:

When it comes to sex, I also felt that I had more ability each time to communicate my knowledge of the baby to my partner. Our deep connection during lovemaking began to include the baby, too, especially with the last one. This was so wonderful—memories I will always treasure. I was with child and the man I love at the same time, and I felt completely fulfilled.

Lesbian mothers report that alignment in menstrual cycling creates a deep physical empathy in pregnancy that enables both to know the baby intimately. From Jen:

Sex with Anne when she was pregnant was an ever-so-much enhanced version of what we had known before. I felt very connected to the baby. Knowing Anne so well, it was easy to differentiate the baby's energy from hers.

Throughout pregnancy, oxytocin levels continue to rise. Oxytocin initiates Braxton-Hicks contractions, which tone the uterus and prepare it for labor. In large amounts, oxytocin is also shown to cause mood elevation and alleviate depression—perhaps this accounts for the feelings of joy and well-being many women experience at this stage of pregnancy. Take ample amounts of oxytocin, mix with high levels of estrogen, blend with vaginal engorgement, and no wonder women in their second trimester may find themselves sexually insatiable, surprising both themselves and their partners. Jeanine states:

To be perfectly honest, I masturbated almost every day. It felt very natural to me. Jack was worried that sex would hurt the baby, but our doctor told him to forget his fears. My vagina was so pliable— he could put two or three fingers inside me and I still wanted more, more pressure. I felt like I was opening up for the baby, but when I had orgasms my muscles squeezed so tight Jack said it practically hurt.

Let's take a closer look at men's reactions to sex in pregnancy. If a man feels concern about jeopardizing the pregnancy during the first trimester, feeling the baby move in the second may further compound his fear. The average male believes the vagina to be somewhat delicate, and the idea of deep thrusting close to where a baby is developing makes some men squeamish. But there is more.

A surprising number of men struggle with conflicting images of Madonna/Whore, Mother versus the Lover, unable to blend the two and hence uncertain of how to relate to their pregnant partner sexually. That a woman nurturing new life might also be blatantly lustful and erotic is a powerful merger of two culturally disparate views of femininity. Not only for the outright misogynist deeply at odds with his feminine side but even for the ordinary guy who up to this point had no idea that such a configuration was possible, there is a strong likelihood of sexual inhibition or shutdown.

What is a woman to do if this occurs? Perhaps her care provider can reassure the father, or refer him to a support group or to individual counseling. Deeply ingrained beliefs of this kind are not easy to change, so the situation may not readily improve. For this and many other reasons, women need the support of one another, sharing frank discussion along with body-affirming activities like dance or exercise. Although it may seem odd at first, singing with others is also helpful; it frees the heart, opens the throat, and releases oxytocin. There is a recognized neuromuscular association between the mouth and the vagina: If one is tight, so will the other be.

In many cultures, both today and throughout history, pregnant women have regularly practiced some sort of ritual dance. Contrary to popular belief, belly dancing was not developed to please or seduce men, but rather to support and reinforce the efforts of women in labor. The movements of the dance—the rolling hips and undulating belly—tend naturally to occur during labor in women free of inhibitions. A circle of dancing women must have helped to remind the mother how to let go, at the same time echoing her emotional and physical responses in a deeply bonding experience for all. Where, in our institutionalized birthing system, might we find the privacy and support to do the same?

To return to the issue of Mother/Lover role conflict, some women feel this too and may manifest it either by avoiding sex or by wanting to focus exclusively on the baby. Resulting problems may be considerable, as disrupted intimacy in a rapidly changing relationship can breed estrangement. In my practice, I remind women of the sexual nature of birth and use that as a reference point to encourage them to stay as sexually open as possible. If the woman is heterosexual, I suggest she experiment with positions like side-lying or being on top, which gives her more control over the depth of penetration and rate of thrusting. Labor is, after all, an intensely physical experience; the estimated caloric output of the first birth is equivalent to that of a fifty-mile hike! And it involves the same kind of emotional surrender as spontaneous orgasm. (For more on this, see my book *Orgasmic Birth: Your Guide to a Safe, Satisfying and Pleasurable Birth Experience.*)

An important aside about physical and sexual abuse: Now that support is available, more and more women are becoming aware of forgotten or repressed experiences. For many, the emotional vulnerability of pregnancy may trigger recollections that are doubly difficult to handle if parents or other relatives were involved, and the accompanying sorrows and fears may interfere with the primary relationship. But believe me, it is better to bring these to the surface while pregnant than to have them arise and interfere with labor or mothering. Precisely because pregnancy is such a heightened state, body-based deep therapies like hypnotherapy or Eye Movement Desensitization and Reprocessing (EMDR) are especially suited for reactivating and healing the past.

Other psychological barriers to intimacy may involve anxieties about money, role changes, and security. Any woman who finds herself at a sexual impasse while pregnant should make every effort to find assistance.

Here's a relevant account from Mariann:

I went to a woman's psychotherapy conference while pregnant and took a workshop on sexual abuse. I didn't even know why I was there, really—just for the info, I thought. We went around the room with introductions, and after the first few heart-wrenching accounts, I felt somewhat out of place. But after a time, I remem-

bered something that happened to me as a child, something I'd completely blocked out. I guess I thought it was no big deal—I was fondled by a conductor on a train when I was twelve—but that day, I relived all of my shame and confusion. I learned that women tend to minimize these experiences, even though they have a lot of impact. Just being aware of what happened to me shed light on certain aspects of my personality and the way I am with sex. Being pregnant, I felt open enough to make some changes.

No matter what a woman's personal challenges, midpregnancy is a time for integration, one in which to find stability and prepare for the changes ahead.

This, or early in the third trimester, is also an opportune time for a ritual celebration of the pregnancy and forthcoming birth. Increasingly, women in our culture are honored with a special ceremony that is more in-depth than the conventional baby shower. In Native-American traditions, a Blessingway is performed for every pregnant woman/couple. (See the boxed section below for ideas for a contemporary "Birthingway" celebration.)

The Birthingway*

The Birthingway, which has its roots in Native-American traditions, is a rite to prepare the mother-to-be to surrender to the mysteries of labor and birth. It is a powerful ceremony honoring the pregnant woman's strength and beauty as life-bringer.

Birth rituals are intended to help parents accept a new person into their midst, but they also strengthen the ties that bind us together in community. In the Sudan, each pregnant woman is honored in a ceremony similar to Native-American traditions. Her hair is hennaed, braided, and scented, she wears a special bracelet and leather thong around her

Reprinted from *The Women's Wheel of Life* by Elizabeth Davis and Carol Leonard   (cont'd.)

waist for protection. She lies on a ceremonial mat of palm leaf stems, and her relatives gather around to rub her belly with handfuls of millet porridge: vitamin rich and symbolic of regeneration. In the Mansi tradition, women assist the expectant mother by ritual preparation of birch-bark cradles, special coverlets of swan skin, and pillows of deer fur twice the size of the mother's hand: Once these are ready, they begin work on a reed mattress on which the new mother will sit and sleep for a certain number of days following the birth. Regardless of cultural specifics, the common purpose of a prenatal ceremony is to empower the mother as her time draws near, and to replace fear with affirmations of her sacredness as the gateway for new life.

Birthingways of today are basically gatherings of the mother's closest women friends and relatives, who bring gifts to honor her and her baby. They may wish to create ritual space by smudging with sage or cedar, or may simply choose to sit in a circle and talk, sharing words of wisdom regarding the challenges of motherhood, or perhaps a favorite anecdote regarding birth or child rearing. The mother's hair may then be combed and adorned with feathers, ribbons and shells, her crown bedecked with flowers. Some mothers save these ornaments and use them to make mobiles to hang above the crib. Traditionally, the mother's feet are bathed in herbal teas and rubbed dry with cornmeal (known as the "Santo Domingo" foot rub, this feels heavenly). Bathing and rubbing the mother's feet signify the wish that she will successfully walk the holy path of labor and birth.

All in the circle may then unite by lightly looping a length of red yarn one-by-one around their wrists to symbolize the umbilical cord connection each had to her own mother. A bowl with red-stained eggs (dyed in beet juice, a tradition

(cont'd.)

at Birthingways) can then be passed around the circle, and each woman in turn may speak three blessings: one for the mother, one for the baby, and one for the global community of women. The mother may also be given poetry and song as gifts. Sometimes she is presented with a bundle or pouch of sacred objects.

When it is time to open the circle, the red yarn is cut so that each woman can keep a bracelet around her wrist to hold the mother in her thoughts until she has had her baby. The eggs blessed in the circle are usually buried outside in a special place, where the placenta might later be buried with a tree or rose bush planted above it. (Women who birth in hospital can, by the way, request that their placenta be given to them to take home.)

In creating these rites, it is most important that we stay flexible, letting the personality of the mother be the basis of design. Another simple format involves gathering for the purpose of making a birth garment for her to wear during her labor, such as an oversized T-shirt decorated with fabric pens, stitchery, sequins, etc. As they make the garment, the women can sing or tell stories about birth. At the same time, they may also wish to make a small garment for the baby. Or they could gather to make a quilt, each of them creating their own squares in advance, then assembling them together.

A simple gesture in the Apache tradition is to present the mother with a cornucopia full of fruits, candy, nuts, and money to symbolize abundance in the four life stages of infancy, childhood, adulthood, and old age.

Whatever form it takes, the ceremony is always followed by feasting and levity. At this point, men may also join the party. This is not to say the father can't have his own ritual celebration: Earlier, while the mother was circling with the

(cont'd.)

women, his male friends and relations might have taken him aside to offer their own anecdotes and words of wisdom on parental responsibilities. But since birth takes place in the mother's body, it is crucial that the Birthingway be centered on her. As it concludes, she should feel blessed by her loved ones, and infused with love and courage.

The Third Trimester

By overview: The first trimester represents initiation into pregnancy; the second, integration and equilibrium; and the third, completion and transition to birth and parenting. Sexuality is often disrupted in the third trimester by the physical discomforts of carrying extra weight. Sleep may be sporadic as comfortable positions become harder to find, although side-lying with pillows between the legs and under the belly can help. Heartburn is common, caused both by the uterus compressing the stomach and by progesterone softening the esophageal valve so that stomach acids rise upward; thus a woman may find that the only way she can sleep is propped upright. And she may need to urinate several times nightly because of increased pressure against her bladder. None of this is particularly conducive to amour, but the midday rendezvous, or other creative solutions, can help.

Additionally, pelvic cartilage is softened considerably in the third trimester by both progesterone and estrogen, so that ordinary pressure on the pubic bone becomes uncomfortable. Many women long to feel their partner on top of them, or dream of sleeping on their stomach. These longings, combined with the inconvenience of interrupted sleep, promote readiness to give up pregnancy and get on with labor, simultaneously preparing a woman for the challenges of caring for her newborn.

Backache is another major complaint at this time, as the enlarged uterus greatly distends the abdominal muscles and pulls the back out of alignment. Rocking the pelvis on hands and knees, or while standing or sitting, helps tremendously. Of course, pelvic rocking comes naturally with lovemaking, as does increased circulation, which can soothe and heal the lower back as well.

Emotionally, these are trying times, with mixed feelings in relationships. Sometimes a woman wants to cling to her partner and hold back time, aware that the baby will soon be out in the world/ in the middle of the bed, and nothing will ever be the same again. Sometimes she wants the privacy just to be with the baby, trying to get to know it as well as she can before it is born, so that sex seems extraneous or more for her partner than for herself. Especially when she is thinking of the challenges ahead and her ongoing need for support, a woman may become demanding, moody, or fearful. Other times, she will feel fully confident, excited by the future, and ready to make love to her partner with abandon.

Hormones are largely responsible for this spectrum of response, as they are once again on the move, shifting erratically in preparation for birth. In the last week or so, a drop in progesterone as a precursor to labor can lead to loss of water weight and a feeling of lightness and well-being. Substances called prostaglandins (fatty acids found in the brain, lungs, kidneys, and prostate gland, as well as in seminal and menstrual fluids) increase at term and may be responsible for labor's onset, although the fetus also releases prostaglandins as its brain matures. Prostaglandins soften the cervix and stimulate uterine contractions. Oxytocin also stimulates uterine activity but is less critical in initiating labor than in promoting its progress.

This is why many care providers now encourage intercourse at term, especially if the baby is overdue. Seminal fluid is extremely high in prostaglandins and may thus trigger labor (a substitute may be found in evening primrose oil, which has a similar effect when rubbed gently on the cervix). Sheila Kitzinger, author of *Woman's Experience of Sex* and numerous books on pregnancy, recommends the following sexual technique for getting labor going: She advises a woman to make love on her back, well supported by pillows under her hips, her partner kneeling between her legs, her ankles on his shoulders to allow for the deepest penetration. After he ejaculates, she stays with hips elevated for at least fifteen minutes, so that prostaglandins may be well absorbed by the cervix. Nipple stimulation every ten minutes or so can also help by prompting the release of oxytocin and resulting uterine activity. This technique replicates the medical practice of using prostaglandin suppositories to "ripen" the cervix, followed by an intravenous Pitocin (synthetic oxytocin) drip to induce contractions. Given the choice, most women would probably choose the nonmedical approach, both to avoid the intrusion of technology and to enhance intimacy as labor begins.

Labor and Birth

◎

As labor starts, pregnancy is ending. Many women feel sadness at this, especially if it is to be the last baby or if the pregnancy itself has been especially fulfilling. Others may feel trepidation with the dawning realization that the only way out of labor is through it. Fortunately, women tend to experience a burst of energy at labor's onset, caused by a peak in estrogen and the added effects of oxytocin.

Is childbirth really a sexual event? How can it be, when it's reputed to be so painful? And if birth is sexual in the usual sense, how do women cope in impersonal hospital settings, surrounded by relative strangers?

Let's consider these questions one at a time. Birth as a sexual event—however can we doubt it? After all, it is an intensely physical experience centered in a woman's vagina. In fact, the entire pelvic area is highly stimulated in labor: not just the vagina but the clitoris, rectum, anus, and the supporting tissues and musculature. We can compare the sensations of labor contractions to those of strong menstrual cramps, but with one important difference. Contractions come in waves; they build up steadily instead of taking hold abruptly. Women who have learned to cope with menstrual cramps by relaxing, staying loose and letting go, have a distinct advantage in labor. And here we find parallels to sexual intercourse. Particularly when sex is very passionate and forceful, there may be moments of discomfort with deep thrusting and intense pelvic movement, particularly if the cervix is being hit directly or the uterus is being jolted against the intestines. Relaxation, rhythmic breathing, and a change of position can help a woman ease through these sensations without losing momentum as she would if she tightened up or shut down emotionally. Especially with orgasm, the ability to surrender and diffuse sensation throughout the body is critical.

Deep relaxation, surrender, letting go: When midwives are asked to disclose the secret of giving birth with relative ease, these are the words we choose. More than metaphors for coping, these responses are based on physiological imperatives, as we will see in the following sections. We will also look closely at how environment affects the spontaneity of the birth process.

First-Stage Labor

During the first stage of labor, the cervix dilates fully to allow the baby to pass through the vagina and into the world. The cervical opening, or os, is ordinarily closed or stretches only a fingertip's worth: Now it will dilate to a circle of about 10 cm in diameter.

In early labor, up to about 4 cm dilation, contractions may be scarcely noticeable. They may feel more like waves of pelvic warmth "with an edge" than painful cramping. So how about making love during early labor? Considering the link between sex and oxytocin, this is quite a good idea. A caution, though: Once the waters have broken, vaginal penetration should be avoided as it may cause infection. Otherwise, sex in early labor relaxes the pelvis, gets the hormones pumping, and eases both partners into an intimate and relaxed state conducive to ready progress. Especially if labor is prolonged in the early phase, sex may be just the thing to move it along (nothing wrong with masturbation, either).

Some women feel like staying just shy of orgasm; others do not. Celine reports:

Just being close with our clothes off, being caressed, helped me relax a lot and take the contractions in stride. I don't know why, but kissing was especially good! Even though my partner eventually came inside me, I felt more like taking it easy than focusing on orgasm.

Kissing and letting go—remember the neuromuscular association between mouth and vagina? In her wonderful book *Spiritual Midwifery*, Ina May Gaskin tells of one couple she directed to kiss in a certain way: the woman with her lips on top, spread out over her partner's. This led to a tangible shift in labor's intensity and very rapid progress. As the classic line from this book reminds us, "The same energy that gets the baby in, gets the baby out."[2]

Couples who do make love in early labor are often thrilled to discover a dimension in lovemaking never before experienced. Particularly when attending home births, I have definitely learned my lesson about knocking before entering the labor room: I can think of several times when couples hurriedly pulled their clothes back on or grabbed a blanket, only to have me tell them to go right ahead!

Still, no matter how well a woman has prepared and has eagerly anticipated labor, there may come a time when the going gets rough, as the sensations begin to exceed her expectations. This is the point when preconceptions about what labor will be like and ideas about how to cope and behave must be swept aside for the real thing. In these moments of reckoning, a woman may find that she must go further in letting go, both physically and emotionally, than she ever has before. It dawns on her that labor is bigger than she is, beyond her experience or control. This can be frightening, as it tends to occur fairly early, at just 4 or 5 cm dilation. She may feel that she has already tried everything and still cannot handle it.

Truth is, she's not going to handle or do it as her ordinary self: She must let herself be transformed to find the way. As you may surmise, this is also a time when many women ask for drugs, particularly if they feel unsupported or exposed.

Imagine yourself in the hospital (hardly an intimate environment), struggling with labor sensations much stronger than you expected, and painful the second you tense up or break your concentration. The constant stream of medical personnel in and out of your room makes it nearly impossible to let go and relax. You find yourself afraid, wanting to cry out or move around and change positions, but you just can't; your circumstances are far too inhibiting. Your attendants are sympathetic, but no one is really getting down to your level, looking you in the eye. Though your partner is standing by, she or he also feels afraid and helpless.

Niles Newton, to whom we must be forever grateful for her groundbreaking research on birth, breast-feeding, and sexuality, investigated the importance of environmental factors on the birth of mice. She found that births were longer and more difficult when mice were placed in unfamiliar surroundings, could not smell or see what they were used to, were moved repeatedly during labor, or were placed in clear (as opposed to opaque) cages. Opposite factors of familiar surroundings, privacy, and stability contributed to spontaneous, easy deliveries.[3]

It was Grantly Dick-Read, author of *Childbirth Without Fear*, who first revealed how fear or tension can cause pain and lack of progress in labor. Beginning with the structure of the uterus, which is comprised of an outer layer of longitudinal fibers and an inner layer of circular fibers, he explained that in the absence of fear or tension, oxytocin causes the long fibers not only to contract but also to retract and become shorter, pulling on the inner fibers encircling the cervix and causing dilation. But if a woman is frightened or tense, elevated adrenaline levels shunt blood away from the uterus and cause the circular fibers to become rigid. The two muscle layers then work against each other, and pain results.[4] Similarly, if you are tense or frightened during lovemaking, you are not likely to experience orgasm.

How to avoid all this? Picture yourself in a darkened room with just your partner, the two of you close and in each other's arms, your care provider sitting quietly in the corner, coming over now and then to offer encouragement or check the baby's heart rate, and then retiring to an adjacent area so your privacy is complete. You still have to deal with the pain, both the physical intensity and the psychological shock of "it's not what I expected," but you can speak freely, you can cry, laugh, shout, or do whatever else suits you: It is your experience. (If you are not partnered, you can experience much the same by engaging the services of a doula to support you physically and emotionally.)

The above scenario is typical of home birth, and in rare circumstances, hospital birth. What tends to derail this experience in the hospital is the routine use of interventions, even during normal labor. Once the decision is made for one such intervention, others are likely to follow. For example, when Pitocin is used to speed up labor (whether due to guidelines for progress or for practitioner convenience), contractions may become so unnaturally strong and painful that a woman requires pain relief. If she receives an epidural, a drop in her blood pressure may slow contractions so that more Pitocin is required to keep labor going. But if the uterus is forced beyond its capacity and cannot relax fully between contractions, impaired circulation means less oxygen gets to the baby. This can lead to fetal distress, with the probable conclusion of Cesarean section. We call this the *cascade of interventions*, all too common in birth today.

In fact, one in three births in the United States today is by Cesarean section; this is shocking but not really surprising, considering the scenario above. Some women even request Cesarean birth, believing it to be less threatening and easier to handle than vaginal birth. Little do they know that Cesarean section is major abdominal surgery with long-term health impacts on mother and baby, nor are they told how difficult recovery can be when one must deal with postoperative pain, tend a baby, establish breast-feeding, suffer sleep deprivation, and cope with the sweeping physiological and emotional changes of the postpartum period.

Old medical texts teach that less than 5 percent of births involve complications. Our 33 percent Cesarean rate has mostly iatrogenic causes; that is, those generated by technology, procedure, or practitioner. The fact that our malpractice compensation system does not discriminate between acts of fate and negligence has forced medical practice to be increasingly defensive, based more on the "standard of care" than on what the data show. Under fear of lawsuit, every possible test and procedure is run, no matter how painful or irrelevant to the mother's condition. Add to this our culturally inculcated expectation of perfection, and the high rate of Cesarean birth becomes even more understandable.

The fact remains that birth is a mystery, one that can never be fully circumscribed by technology. Even in the most carefully monitored situations, hemorrhages occur unexpectedly, babies get stuck at the shoulder, cord accidents happen at the last minute, babies and mothers die. The bottom line is that here in the United States, in spite of all our interventions, we have a higher perinatal mortality rate than most countries where birth occurs spontaneously and is frequently attended at home: We rank #30, meaning that 29 countries lose fewer babies than we do.[5] Even worse, accompanying the rise in Cesarean section is increased maternal mortality: In this category, the United States ranks #42.[6] Thus pregnant women must make every effort to see beyond propaganda and marketing in order to make wise decisions regarding who will attend their birth and where it will take place.

In case you are curious about the safety of home birth, in 2005 the *British Medical Journal* (a prestigious and highly selective periodical) published the largest and most reputable study of home birth in North America. (You can access "The CPM 2000 Study," by Ken Johnson and Betty-Anne Daviss, at bmj.com.) In this study of 5,418 planned home births assisted by CPMs (the national credential for midwives trained for home birth), only 12 percent of women transferred to the hospital, and of these, only 4.7 percent had epidural anesthesia, 2.1 percent had an episiotomy, and 3.7 percent gave birth by Cesarean section. No mothers died, and the intrapartum/neonatal mortality rate was 1.7 in 1,000, similar to rates in other studies of low-risk home or hospital birth. Maternal satisfaction rates were high, at 97 percent.[7]

Two more studies in Canada showed similar results. The first, from British Columbia, compared 2,899 home births with registered midwives, 4,604 hospital births with registered midwives, and 5,331 hospital births with physicians. The infant mortality rate for home birth was 0.035 percent; for midwife-assisted births in hospital, 0.057 percent; and for physician-assisted births in hospital, 0.095 percent.[8] The second study, from Ontario, showed no significant difference in perinatal and neonatal mortality in 6,692 women who had planned home births and the same number who had planned hospital births, although rates of serious maternal complications were significantly lower at home.[9]

Returning to the course of labor: Whatever your environment, once you enter the active phase (with contractions long and strong, coming about every five minutes), neurohormones called endorphins flood your bloodstream. These are released with any intense physical activity; you may have experienced them as a "second wind" or "runner's high." With the endorphins kicked in, many women begin to enjoy labor and may even find it an ecstatic experience. One of my clients who was crying and desperate in early labor was smiling and dancing around the room at 9 cm. Not every woman maintains an external focus so far into labor; it depends on how quickly labor is progressing and how strong contractions are. Many women turn inward as they approach full dilation, eyes closed between contractions, and peacefully out of body. Still, there is always the exception, like the woman who laughed, chatted, and ate fried chicken until she was ready to push!

Endorphins are also released with sexual activity and lead to the exquisite feeling of afterglow. However, if pain medications are used during labor, stress perception will be minimal and endorphin release may not occur. Although pain may be nearly obliterated by medication, so too will the ecstatic, transcendent feelings many women report in giving birth naturally.

When my book *Orgasmic Birth: Your Guide to a Safe, Satisfying and Pleasurable Birth Experience* was about to go to print, a last-minute account came in from a mother who found a unique way to alleviate pain and make labor easier. Planning a home birth, she warned her doula in advance that she might hear some unusual sounds coming from the bedroom. Apparently her friends, upon hearing that she wanted an orgasmic birth, had given her a selection of vibrators as shower gifts, and she intended to use them! Having done so, she reported that the only time she felt pain was when she tried going without. Once she was pushing, the vibrators were set aside, but she was thrilled with her experience and happy to share it. Imagine if women having hospital births set up their bedside table with a vibrator in prominent display: Talk about a way to secure some privacy!

The need for privacy in labor is physiologic, for when women feel observed—whether by attendants, technology, or their own analysis—the neocortex is stimulated, adrenaline is released, and oxytocin diminishes. It is rather like being in the midst of lovemaking when suddenly, someone knocks on the door, or (god forbid) opens it. As for the self-observation aspect: You know how hard it is to reach orgasm when worrying about or evaluating your performance? The same is true of making progress in labor.

Unfortunately, hospital standards for labor progress further complicate matters. The expectation that dilation should occur at the rate of a centimeter per hour is unrealistic, in that it is based on the average length of labor, not its usual course. Spontaneous birth typically features phases of several hours when women have no change in dilation, but far from being dysfunctional, these plateaus in progress are times of integrating new levels of sensation or psychological intensity. Once a plateau is past, women often progress very rapidly: as much as 5 cm in less than an hour. This correlates to female sexual response, which also features plateaus. Sheila Kitzinger goes so far as to suggest that medicine has superimposed a male-ejaculatory model on women's variable intensity, multiple-orgasmic birthing nature, and I can't help but agree.[10]

What comes next in the birth process? Even women who have never been pregnant have heard of the transition phase of labor, reputed to be the most difficult of all. Not every woman experiences transition, but for those who do, it occurs between 8 and 10 cm dilation. Physically, the cervix continues to dilate as the baby descends through it and pushes onto the pelvic floor. This results in conflicting prompts to "relax, stay open, surrender," and "push, bear down, get busy!" Just when a woman feels she has finally made peace with completely letting go, she suddenly feels compelled to act. At this, her emotions swing wildly; she may swear at her partner or birth attendants. Hormonally, ongoing rushes of oxytocin are interspersed with surges of adrenaline.

How can these purportedly conflicting hormones work in concert? There are two different types of uterine receptors for adrenaline: beta-inhibitor and alpha-initiator. When dilation gives way to bearing down, adrenaline stimulates the alpha-initiator receptors to help the mother actively participate in birthing her baby. Adrenaline is also a precursor to prostaglandin release (bringing to mind the characteristic burst of energy just before labor starts), and increased prostaglandin levels are thought to be responsible for the bearing-down reflex. Tying human physiology to animal behavior in the wild, physician Michel Odent notes that if threatened in early labor, mothers usually wait until they can safely give birth, but if labor is well advanced or is happening quickly, it is to their advantage to birth as soon as possible.[11]

Odent further notes that the natural release of adrenaline at this point may be accompanied by surges of fear or anxiety. But is adrenaline a precursor to these emotions, or is it the other way around? In either case, if a woman experiences panic, at least she can feel comforted in knowing it is normal. She may have mortal fear, as if fighting for survival. She may cry out or scream. This is in direct contrast to what is taught in most childbirth preparation classes, that women should make only low-pitched sounds lest they tighten up. On the contrary, women left to their own devices often scream or roar as they enter second stage, leaping to their feet or into a crouch with superhuman strength. These same women later revel in the power of this moment. "Those sounds," one recalled, "where were they coming from? Some deep part of me that had never been touched before. They rang in my ears—raw, clear, and unbelievably strong." "I felt so primal," said another, "like some sort of tigress, a jungle queen." For many, this is one of the most sexual moments in giving birth, one that can transform a previously shy or inhibited woman into a powerfully assertive lover.

Second-Stage Labor

To backtrack a bit, we must clarify that although second-stage labor commences with full dilation, some women do not experience the adrenaline surge and urge to push for some time after, especially if the baby is not yet pressing on the pelvic floor. Sometimes, if labor has been long or difficult thus far, the uterus takes a break, contractions stop, and the mother takes a nap! This is known as the "rest and be thankful" phase, after which the urge to push commences. As this gets stronger, pressure begins to build in the vagina. What is this sensation like? Imagine something the size of a grapefruit (the baby's head) pressing hard on all the sensitive areas deep inside you, combined with a downward squeezing urge something like moving your bowels but ten times stronger—a whole-body urge turning you inside out—and you have some idea of the sensory magnitude. No wonder we need a burst of adrenaline to help us through! By this point, the uterus has stretched and thinned in the lower segment, with long fibers retracted to form a mass at the top that pushes the baby downward. It is the uterus that pushes the baby out, not the mother, although her ability to cooperate with her body makes a difference in ease of progress. Second stage can consist of twenty minutes of urges so overwhelming that you can scarcely catch your breath, or it may last several hours with urges of varying length and intensity, sometimes so light you can breathe right through them.

Once again, however, we find medical management at odds with physiology: Hospital staff seem determined in nearly every case to get the baby out as soon as possible. Women are told to draw their legs back forcibly, hold their breath as long as possible, and push their guts out with every contraction. This is rather like trying to force orgasm, riding over the rhythm instead of with it. To put it another way, under which circumstances might you find it easier to have an orgasm: with someone barking orders at you every step of the way, or when free to surrender to your body and let it take you? Most probably, aggressive management of second stage is due to persisting notions that it is dangerous for both mother and baby to let the fetal head "pound the perineum." It may also signify an inculcated fear of the vagina as a dangerous place. In reality, forced, insensitive pushing often causes damage to vaginal tissues, at the same time depriving the baby of oxygen. As demonstrated by researcher and physician Roberto Caldeyro-Barcia, unnaturally long periods of maternal breath-holding lead to fetal acidosis and distress.[12] Again, we see the influence of the male-ejaculatory model on the pushing process, for which the variable-intensity, multiple-orgasmic female model is imminently more suitable.

When a woman in second stage is unfettered by outside direction she will, in fact, breathe very much as she would during sexual excitation and orgasm: up to three times more rapidly than usual, with periods of breath-holding punctuated by gasps, groans, or cries. Women allowed to push their babies out spontaneously often describe birth as orgasmic, speaking of tremendous release, ecstatic rushes of emotion, and overwhelming happiness. I have observed that if women are controlled by others while pushing, they are somewhat inhibited at first with their babies.

For me, the ecstasy of second stage occurred when my uterus and I were working as one, beyond signal and response. In this mode, a woman can literally birth on her own, sensing exactly when she can take more stretch and when to ease up, gently breathing her baby out. Because I had been given a huge episiotomy (a cut to enlarge the birth canal) with my first birth, I was so determined not to tear with the second that I really tuned in during pushing—just closed my eyes and did it from the inside. I could feel everything, the precise contours of my daughter's head as I eased it out, even her little shoulders and body as she whooshed and squiggled through. It was absolutely the most exquisite thing I have felt in my life. Later, my midwives said they wished we had the birth on tape, because I was so perfectly controlled. But for me, control had nothing to do with it, as I wasn't holding back. Beyond attunement, there was union, perfect union.

In sheep, vaginal stimulation has been shown to be a critical factor in bonding. In one study, *nonpregnant* ewes primed with estrogen and progesterone that were vaginally stimulated (by vibrator) responded to newborn lambs with a full range of bonding behaviors. With the same stimulation, ewes that had recently given birth and had already bonded to their own lambs stopped rejective behavior toward foreign lambs and accepted them as their own.[13] Krehbiel and associates found that giving peridural (pelvic floor) anesthetic to birthing ewes, particularly if early in labor, severely altered normal maternal behavior: Seven of the eight first-time mothers failed to show any bonding response in the first half hour. Ewes that had given birth previously responded less dramatically but still showed some effects.[14] Perhaps the choice of epidural anesthesia, which numbs to a greater extent than does peridural, is not as benign as we have been led to believe. I have noticed that once an epidural is administered, a woman becomes more a spectator of her birth than a participant. She is often at a loss as to what to do with her newborn, whereas the unmedicated mother usually responds to her baby passionately, with fiercely protective instincts.

This raises yet another issue, that of vaginal tearing with delivery. Isn't it better to have an episiotomy, rather than being stretched out or torn?

Here we have one of the biggest lies perpetuated by modern obstetrics: that the human vagina is somehow inadequate to the task of birthing and must be surgically enhanced to accomplish it. Most women don't realize that the vagina's surface is covered with ruggae, accordion-like folds of tissue that expand naturally with the hormonal effects of pregnancy. When a woman is relaxed and centered at delivery, not rushed but well supported, she will generally give birth without a scratch, or with abrasions so minor they require no treatment. And despite beliefs to the contrary, episiotomies do not heal better than tears: If a tear does require stitches, its irregular edges mesh together better and close more quickly than the clean-edged episiotomy wound. Finally, it is much easier to regain sexual pleasure and muscle responsiveness after repair of a tear than an episiotomy. Tears frequently skim the surface, but in doing an episiotomy one is obliged to cut deeply through muscle. The result is a wall of scar tissue, often inflexible and numb to sensation for quite some time.

But what about vaginal snugness after birth? How can an area that has been stretched so dramatically ever regain its former tone? Isn't that what the "husband's knot" is for? Talk about disgusting terminology! This excessively tight stitch at the base of the vaginal opening does little more than cause pain and distress with penetration. Pleasurable friction is found less at the opening than from the muscles immediately inside the vagina. Although it is possible to create a tight opening with episiotomy and repair, the scarred portions inside will be rigid, the supporting muscles flaccid, and the entire area dysfunctional for many months. When the vagina is intact after birth, the muscles continue to respond as a unit.

Keep in mind that when a woman is fully aroused, she spontaneously tightens those muscles just inside the vaginal opening, while the back portion of the canal balloons to several inches deeper and wider: nature's design to allow seminal fluid to pool around the cervix. In general, a woman who has birthed spontaneously and has re-toned her vaginal muscles postpartum will be a more responsive and pleasurable partner than one with deep-tissue trauma and repair (at least until healing occurs, which can take a long time).

In the 1950s, when the husband's knot became a standard part of repair technique, women were not taught pelvic-floor exercises (see page 119), and few explored their own musculature for fear of hurting themselves or doing something "dirty." Sexual mores were based on male gratification: Little was known or understood about female sexual response. Times have changed; women are more embodied now, and most have no qualms about putting their fingers inside to help them locate and tone their vaginal muscles. When a woman is in touch this way and plans to give birth without an episiotomy but receives one anyhow, she may feel violated and emotionally traumatized. As one woman, Jan, said of her first birth:

> *I felt I was doing a good job, easing my baby out nicely, when suddenly and for no apparent reason my doctor changed his mind and cut me. I felt defeated, like, "Oh…well, okay, I give up…guess I'm not good enough." I lost all feeling, and he took control.*

I have assisted more than three hundred births and have only had to perform episiotomy five times, each because last-minute fetal distress necessitated immediate delivery. Seldom do women in my practice tear, and if they do, the tear is usually minor and requires no stitches. This is no miracle; it's simply a matter of helping women feel safe enough to let go and tune into their sensations. When women birth in water, there is natural counterpressure to the area. If not in water, hot compresses to the perineum can be a great comfort and offer a sense of containment.

The Birth

At the final moment of crowning, when the widest part of the baby's head stretches the vaginal opening to its maximum, some women love either to look in a mirror or to reach down and touch their little one for the first time. Sometimes this brings a tremendous flood of emotion, and the baby is born in an orgasm of sensation. Most women describe the moment of birthing as the high point of their lives, a physical and emotional pinnacle. All the waiting and wondering, all hopes and fears are finally unleashed and allowed to rush forward as the baby swooshes out and utters its first cry.

Mothers often catch their own babies in water birth, but if the mother is not in water, she can still reach down and lift her baby up when it is still partly inside her: something she will never forget. The baby is wet, warm, incredibly fragile yet surprisingly strong. It smells sweetly of birth. She touches its little hands and feet and then finds herself falling into its eyes, seeing the faces of relatives and ancestors, feeling past and future unite. Birth is a stunning victory for a woman, especially when she has retained her power and knows she has given it her all.

Birth Is a Blood Mystery

The real truth is that birth is a mystery, one by which we grow and learn exponentially as compared to ordinary life lessons. Here is a tale of our heritage as birthing women.

◎   ◎   ◎

Once, women walked the world in beauty and confidence. They were revered and kept safe by their communities. When such a woman came to her time to give birth, she had already seen the births of siblings or other relatives, or had assisted her close women friends. She had no question of her body's worth and power, no

(cont'd.)

fear of rape or abuse. Her menarche had been cause for great celebration; she was guided through this rite of passage with ritual and song—and it was deeply joyous! Now she would explore the unknown once again, but within the container of meaning given by her culture, supported by a circle of women of all ages, and guided by the midwives.

She was nourished well as labor began, bathed and adorned. As her pains became stronger, she began her journey to the birth hut. Along her way were a series of upright poles she could use for support; she moved to the next only when labor dramatically intensified, so that by the time she reached the birth hut she was nearly ready. There her circle of supporters surrounded her more closely, dancing sensually, chanting and smiling, touching her as needed. The passion of birth took her completely, and she surrendered to its power. As she did so, pain became interspersed with ecstasy, and she sank into blissful rest between each contraction, her spirit traveling far and wide. Soon she felt urges to push and became more upright, held and encouraged, gentle hands brushing her hair back from her forehead. She had never felt so open, so boundless and vulnerable, yet so strong. Her baby moving down inside her brought new sensations, so much intensity, yet still she could clearly feel its exquisite form. She gave way completely, panting and surging, and her baby glided out into the world onto the bed of soft grass beneath her. What wonder, what beauty, what joy! She reached down to touch, and slowly took the baby up with her hands and into her arms. Her placenta was soon birthed, handled carefully that its ritual and healing powers might be preserved.

In the weeks that followed, she and her partner were fed and cared for by the women elders. Each day, and for long periods of time, she was attended by these women, who saw to her personal needs, chatted with her about community affairs, and instructed

(cont'd.)

her in her new role. A fire was kept burning to keep her living space warm enough for her to be without clothes, so she might readily heal and breast-feed with ease. After a period of six weeks, she and the baby were officially welcomed to the community. When her best friend gave birth a year later, she was at her side with confidence and encouragement.

In the next chapter, we will explore the tender and tempestuous postpartum period, and look at how sexual identity and expression are affected and transformed by the presence of a newborn.

CHAPTER 5

Sex *after the* Baby Comes

The postpartum period is defined as a minimum of six weeks and a maximum of three years after giving birth. This is undoubtedly one of the sweetest and most challenging times of a woman's life. It has wisely been said that the exhilaration of pregnancy and birth are but preparation for the grueling adjustments to be made postpartum. I often tell women that the first six weeks of caring for a newborn is the hardest work they will ever do. The changes involved in adding a member to the family are far from minor, and the stress of it all may well lead a woman to wonder whether there is sex after birth.

The Recovery Process

With a little patience and creativity, sex usually comes back better than ever, even though modifications are called for at first. To truly understand sexuality during this phase, we must look at the physical process of recovery as well as that of lactation.

In the first few moments following the birth, fresh spurts of oxytocin are released to contract the uterus and shear off the placenta. As the baby begins to nurse, nipple stimulation triggers more oxytocin release, which shrinks the uterus down to the size of a grapefruit. Adrenaline (present in large amounts at the moment of birth to prompt alertness and bonding between the mother and her newborn) diminishes so that both are able to rest. Over the next ten days or so, continued release of oxytocin will contract the uterus back to its pre-pregnancy size.

When a woman breast-feeds, oxytocin levels soar higher according to the frequency of nursing, which in the first few weeks may occur as often as every hour or two. The extra boost serves to contract and tone the upper vaginal area (or vault), a process that takes place much more slowly in women who bottle-feed.

Milk production is initiated in part by the hormone prolactin, which is released when estrogen and progesterone levels drop with birth. Continued milk production depends on stimulation of the breasts: The more the baby sucks, the more milk the mother will produce, as long as she has adequate rest, food, and drink. Letdown of milk with each nursing is triggered by oxytocin via nipple stimulation. Oxytocin also increases blood flow to the breasts, causing them to radiate heat so the baby is literally bathed in warmth.

What does letdown feel like? For most women, it's very pleasurable. It begins with tingling sensations in the breasts, followed by tightening as they fill, and then strong physical urges for release. We have, I think, a ready correlation here to what men experience with arousal. There is an imperative need to be partnered that accompanies letdown: A mother experiencing it wants her baby *now*.

It seems obvious that breast-feeding is a sexual experience. Sometimes, uterine and vaginal contractions caused by oxytocin even lead to orgasm. Unless a woman has deep inhibitions, breast-feeding is at the very least physically fulfilling, with surges of warmth and wellbeing that encompass body and soul. And the experience is mutual: The baby responds with love and desire, its little hands stroke the breast, its toes curl rhythmically, its body presses forward (as it gets older). Just as making love bonds emotionally healthy adults together, breast-feeding bonds mother and child. In fact, suckling at the breast triggers the release of oxytocin in the newborn, which not only helps stabilize its mood but also facilitates digestion. We are little accustomed to thinking of babies as having sexual needs, but to a certain extent, they do. Close to our most basic definition of sexual desire is the physical and emotional urge for intimacy that is with us from birth.

Niles Newton and Charlotte Modahl found that mood changes occurring with lovemaking and orgasm are very much like those that accompany breast-feeding. Their study showed that women who bottle-feed have higher levels of anxiety, stress, depression, and guilt than mothers who breast-feed.[1] According to the research of E. B. Thoman and associates, lactating women show a suppression of adrenaline release (and accompanying neurological activity) in response to trauma.[2] The release of oxytocin through breast-feeding appears to be a biological perk to help women buffer stress and make it through the emotional and physical challenges of this phase.

Postpartum adjustment is indeed more than a matter of restoring pelvic anatomy and establishing breast-feeding. Remember the many physiologic changes of pregnancy mentioned in Chapter 4: increased blood volume, increased thyroid and kidney function, decreased vascular tension, slowed digestion, and so on. In the first few weeks postpartum, these body functions shift back to pre-pregnant norms. But this is hardly a smooth, even process; rather, it is fitful and erratic. Hormones ebb, flow, and only gradually stabilize. The resulting hot flashes and cold spells, night sweats, and mood swings make this a biologically and emotionally charged period for women and their families (similar to menopause).

Emotional Change and Adjustment

◎

Distinguishing the hormonally induced mood swings that occur postpartum from more serious psychological problems can be something of a challenge in our culture. That we treat the new mother as though nothing has changed, expecting her to be back on her feet and in charge of her affairs in a matter of days, is the height of denial. In nearly every society but ours, continuous support is provided to all new mothers during their "lying-in" period, with their only obligation to stay in bed and focus on the baby. This may be for six weeks or just ten days, but in any case, mothering the mother helps her bond more deeply with her baby and recover more completely. The better she feels, the more easily she will integrate her new role. As she learns to honor the needs of her child as well as her own, both benefit greatly. Care of new mothers assures survival of the species, but more than that, it positively affects quality of life for all of us.

Postpartum customs of Native-American and Indonesian cultures specifically involve the use of heat, as new mothers are considered to be "open" from birthing and therefore susceptible to chill and loss of energy. A fire may be built near or even under the mother's bed so she may nurse spontaneously, remain unclothed, and feel at ease. Far from the numbing isolation mothers commonly experience in our society, women of these cultures are surrounded by female peers and extended family who feed and counsel them, joke with them, and marvel at the miracle of their newborn child. In the Philippines, the new mother is believed to be in such a state of grace that should she die in the first forty days postpartum, her soul will automatically go to heaven.

When a woman is not well cared for at this time, there are complex, often long-term effects on her body, personality, and sexuality. Although oxytocin has the ability to buffer stress, it has its limits. If a woman is forced out of bed or back to work too soon, overproduction of adrenaline will derail her recovery. As Newton observes, "Oxytocin reflexes can be severely inhibited by environmental disturbances, emotional upset or pain."[3] Thus the "Amazon concept" of postpartum recovery can be nothing but myth: Women never did give birth in the bush and jump immediately back on their horses, unless their survival depended on it. To put it another way: Our scandalously high incidence of postpartum depression in the United States has frustrated biological needs at its root. Without sufficient rest, postpartum recovery is grueling and prolonged. And sex is on the far back burner.

The same cultural ideology that deems it appropriate to abandon the new mother may further challenge her changing identity. In assuming her new role, she is bound to experience loss, some of it painful. Single friends may abandon her, finding it impossible to relate to what she is experiencing. Her primary relationship has already been altered: Now it may become somewhat strained. She herself is inextricably changed; her old routines and ways of handling the most basic tasks no longer work. Privacy seems a thing of the past, at least for the time being. If she takes maternity leave, she may experience a loss of income and change in her standard of living. And finally, what should be at most a temporary loss of energy and resourcefulness may become permanent unless she receives assistance. Without it, chronic fatigue may lead to depression. New mothers are fragile, vulnerable, and impressionable: Well-meaning but misguided advice sinks deep, and criticism is not easily forgotten.

More than anything else, giving birth makes clear that control in life is an illusion. Ideally, a woman's experience of making this discovery is positive, even exhilarating; if not, her self-esteem may be diminished. This is also a cause of depression. One of my most critical tasks in caring for clients postpartum is to help them debrief their birth experience. Women sometimes express anxiety about their performance in labor as early as day three, and they may call again in tearful panic over the next few weeks for more discussion, more reassurance. This is particularly true if the birth has been difficult or the outcome disappointing. Certainly the course of acceptance will be rocky if there are problems with the baby's health or physical condition. But a woman can have a lovely, healthy baby and still be devastated by her birth experience. Until very recently, women were denied the right to grieve their birth disappointments; as my mother was told when she complained to her doctor about the indignities she suffered at the hands of hospital staff, "If the cake is good, eat it!" She told me this just days after my own traumatic first birth, and it remains one of the fateful moments in my life when I said to myself, "No, that is not enough, I am worth more than that, women are worth more than that!"

Yet another aspect of a mother's recovery has to do with whether bonding was disrupted. Much research has been done on this subject, most of it showing damaging effects if mother and baby are separated for more than moments during the first few hours, especially immediately after birth. Animals thus separated respond in classic, predictable ways: The newborn will bond with whatever is available—even another species, or something mechanical—and the mother will reject her young when later reintroduced. This is potent genetic programming meant to ensure survival, and when it is disrupted in the human sphere, a woman feels rather like Humpty Dumpty: Who can put the pieces back together again? And if she stays in the hospital for more than a few hours, bonding may be further disrupted by nurses who feel obliged (or may choose) to begin caring for the baby: dressing it, changing its diaper, comforting it in her presence. All these are critical tasks the mother needs to handle so that she may awaken her natural maternal instincts and develop her own foundation for caregiving.

It is both curious and disappointing that one of our leading feminist thinkers, Gloria Steinem, traced the problem of low self-esteem no further back than to early childhood. She acknowledged that "as infants and small children, we cannot possibly earn our welcome in this world," but she failed to link low self-esteem to our experience at birth.[4] She stressed the importance of "honoring the wisdom of the body," and yet seemed unaware of how deeply this wisdom can be violated by a traumatic birth experience. If birth is perceived as negative and/or bonding is impaired, a chain reaction of missed communications between mother and baby may make efforts to develop the relationship frustrating and exceedingly difficult.

Breast-feeding provides a critical way to reestablish bonds that were broken with a difficult birth. Counseling is increasingly available for women who need help with this. Fortunately, in spite of the crucial importance of bonding at birth, we human females are distinct from other mammals in that we have the intelligence to deliberately re-create our bonds with our young. This is far from easy, but it can be done.

What does all this have to do with postpartum sexuality? At the most basic level, the key to sexual happiness in this phase is found in the mother's integration and self-respect. She must recognize her new role, work out her birth experience, acknowledge her changed identity, and deepen her attachment to her baby. If she is able to do all this, she will generally return to her intimate relationship with enthusiasm. There are a few practical concerns regarding sex at this time (addressed later in this chapter), but ultimately, sex postpartum is not about timing and technique any more than it is at any other phase of a woman's life. The reason many guidebooks take this focus is that dealing with the underlying issues is daunting, to say the least. But if the only advice we can offer a new mother concerned about her sex life is to make love in the afternoon when the baby sleeps, she is apt to feel that even her sexuality has been pared down to practicality—that it, too, was lost when she gave birth.

There is ample evidence that a good bond between mother and baby makes for better sex. Masters and Johnson found that breast-feeding women had a higher level of sexual interest than bottle-feeding mothers. As a group, they sought as rapid a return as possible to sexual activity with their partners.[5]

But the data is contradictory. Other studies show a marked decline in sexual interest among breast-feeding mothers. This is attributed to the hormone prolactin, which is known to diminish sex drive.

Oxytocin can counter the effects of prolactin, but one study showed that the amount of oxytocin in the systems of breast-feeding women is highly variable. Mothers who nursed for long stretches tended to have the highest levels overall, and also experienced spikes from time to time.[6]

Yet another substance, a neurotransmitter known as dopamine, modifies the effects of prolactin. Dopamine is the "feel good" hormone associated with desire: It causes us to perceive and pursue pleasure. Sexual activity increases our levels of both oxytocin and dopamine.

What does all this mean? The data suggest that although prolactin has a subduing effect on the sex drive, women may be able to counteract this both by nursing their babies on demand and by making love. In other words, sex itself can be a remedy for sexual disinterest. You may have already found this to be true empirically: If you have ever gone for long periods without sex, you probably got quite comfortable without it, but once you resumed sexual activity, you couldn't wait for the next encounter. Perhaps while breast-feeding we must make an effort to have sex in order to keep this cycle going, especially since prolactin will continue to intervene until weaning has occurred.

Maintaining optimal health is critical too. This means eating plenty of fresh, nourishing food, as breast-feeding mothers require approximately 500 more calories a day than nonpregnant women. Supplements taken during pregnancy should be continued, with stress-reduction techniques utilized on a regular basis.

Practicalities of Postpartum Sex

◎

Now we are ready to discuss the more concrete details of postpartum sexuality. Especially at first, women are greatly concerned about their internal healing and potential vulnerability with lovemaking, particularly if they have had stitches and there is tenderness or stiffness at the site of injury.

Physicians commonly have women return for a checkup at six weeks postpartum to assess the healing of the perineum and make recommendations for contraception, as appropriate. But most women are told little or nothing of how to care for the perineum in the interim, or what to watch for that might signal infection, such as inflammation or swelling. Pain is an important signal too, but it may go unnoticed if a woman is taking painkillers during the first few days—the most critical time for healing.

I suggest that women use cold packs for twenty-four hours to reduce swelling, then switch to sitz baths several times daily using hot water with selected herbs. Nothing speeds healing faster than heat, and soaking is far superior to topical application as it more deeply stimulates circulation. Fresh ginger is a good addition to the solution as it helps relieve the itching that often occurs as stitches dissolve and the skin heals.

Here is how I recommend that women take a sitz bath: Grate a three-to-four-inch piece of ginger into a large pot of water, simmer twenty minutes, strain, and divide into two portions. Save one for later in the day, and dilute the first with water in a sitz bath unit (a special plastic tub that fits over the toilet seat, available at most pharmacies). After soaking for twenty minutes, thoroughly dry the perineum and expose to air or sunlight for another ten minutes before putting on a fresh pad (or use a hair dryer to speed the process). If the perineum feels at all sticky, you can use aloe vera gel to dry and soothe the tissues. Avoid vitamin E or other oil-based ointments until the skin is healed over, as these tend to keep edges from closing.

Despite the six-week ban on intercourse/penetration, some women go ahead with it before returning to their practitioner for permission. Sometimes this is fine; sometimes the experience is so fraught with anxiety and discomfort that it is both worrisome and disappointing. Why the time limit at all? Ordinarily, it takes ten days for the uterus to return to normal size and for the cervix to close securely, with a minimum of two weeks for all bleeding to stop. Sex during this time can increase bleeding or may lead to uterine infection. Stitches are a major contraindication to sex in the first few weeks, as they take a week or so to dissolve and at least two more to heal. If you had stitches, you really should be checked before having sex, even if it means scheduling an appointment earlier than your practitioner expects or recommends.

Most women are anxious about sex after giving birth. Preliminary self-massage can help, particularly to areas with scar tissue. The wall-like ridge characteristic of episiotomy can be softened and relaxed with thumb or finger pressure, using a little oil (just make sure to wash your hands before handling the baby or breast-feeding). When scarring is extensive, evening primrose oil (found in health-food stores) may significantly help to reduce it. Due to decreased estrogen postpartum, vaginal lubrication may also pose a problem during sex. Water-based lubricating jelly is best, as excess oil can clog delicate vaginal tissues and glands.

Estrogen production and the return of the monthly cycle will occur spontaneously if a mother stops breast-feeding or may gradually resume as she introduces solid foods and the baby nurses less often. There are exceptions, though. Some women nurse their babies (or even toddlers) just once or twice a day and still do not resume their normal cycle. Others may nurse exclusively and have milk in abundance, yet start menstruating as early as six weeks postpartum. The reasons for this discrepancy are uncertain. A number of my clients have observed that sexual activity in the first few weeks postpartum seemed to cause them to start menstruating within the next month. No harm in this; certainly, a woman's sex life will benefit. But babies tend to be fussier when their mothers are menstruating, and PMS can be especially trying if combined with sleep deprivation and fatigue.

If adequately repaired and cared for, the perineum should be fully healed at six weeks no matter how extensive the damage. I recently saw a woman (not my client) who was experiencing pain and bleeding with intercourse seven months after perineal repair! She had been back to see her doctor, who offered little assistance (unfortunately, he was also a relative, so she hesitated to seek a second opinion). As I suspected, she had been sewn up too tightly with the husband's knot. Even gentle pressure to the area caused bleeding, as the skin tore ever so slightly apart. Both she and her partner were frustrated and miserable, and eventually, she had reconstructive surgery. But other women who have seen me for this problem report spontaneous resolution with application of evening primrose oil to the perineum, massaged in thoroughly twice a day.

Bleeding without pain is normal for up to six weeks, but it should be fairly light from three weeks on. It may increase temporarily with intense physical activity, indicating a need for more rest. The first lovemaking may also cause some bleeding afterward, which is perfectly normal. But bleeding that persists past six weeks could indicate that placental fragments have been retained or that overproliferation of the endometrium has occurred. If there is any doubt, see your care provider.

A major concern heterosexual women have about resuming sex is whether they will have sufficient vaginal tone to satisfy their partner. Some tone is usually lost with the birth, although breast-feeding naturally helps to restore it. Pelvic-floor exercises can be resumed as early as the first day postpartum. These aren't particularly easy at first, but they may feel more natural and effective if done while breast-feeding (linking them to a particular activity also makes it easier to remember to do them).

There are three basic pelvic-floor exercises that I recommend. The first tones the vault of the vagina: It is known as the elevator exercise. To do this, relax your muscles completely, then draw them up to the first "floor" and then to the second "floor," for five floors altogether. Hold at each floor for as many seconds as you can, and once your reach the "top," let your muscles down again floor-by-floor, holding at each for as many seconds as you can until you reach the "basement."

The second exercise tones the sidewalls of the vagina and fine-tunes tone in the vault. To do this, relax your vagina completely, and then pull upward with a longitudinal stroking motion, as if you were caressing a soft fruit and squeezing out the juice.

The third exercise tones the bulbocavernosus muscle near the vaginal opening. Again, relax completely, and then quickly contract low in the vagina with quick, snapping movements. Do as many repetitions as you can, increasing these daily. If you are unsure of what you are doing or whether you are making progress, put your fingers inside and find out. These movements are sacred to both Tantric and Kundalini traditions, whereby women initiate the flow of sexual energy up the spine to experience bliss and enlightenment. These movements also occur naturally with orgasm, thus sex itself is a great way to re-tone the vagina.

Here are several accounts of first sex postpartum that serve to illustrate both the awkwardness and the transformation possible at this time. From Tessa:

> *John and I had been through so much with the birth, which we planned for home but ended up having in the hospital. I had complications, but I managed to give birth without needing a Cesarean. Then we had to stay in the hospital because of concerns for our son, and my husband was totally drawn into taking care of everything. He was down in the nursery when they needed to do tests, talking to the staff, protecting the baby, and bringing him right back to me. When we got home we were utterly exhausted, but that very night we made love. I knew I shouldn't—it was only the third day—but we couldn't help it, we had to reunite, the urge was irresistible. It was, I think, the most intimate and explosive sex we've ever had—it just burst from both of us. We had been so close in pregnancy, and we really reached deep for each other to get back to ourselves and heal what happened with the birth. I had a little bleeding after, but it was worth it.*

From Julia:

> *I love Maria more than ever after the birth, to be with her and cuddle with the baby is just the best! We waited a couple weeks until she felt okay—she didn't have stitches or anything, and it was*

lovely to be able to feel inside her again. I was a bit tentative at first,
but I knew she would be honest with me as we went along.

And from Christine:

I waited a full four weeks, and Jarred was at his limit. I hadn't
been to the doctor yet, but I'd been looking in a mirror and feeling
around, and everything seemed fine. Well, when he got inside me
it felt so different that I think it shocked us both. The part that
had stitches felt numb and stiff, and the rest of me felt all loose
and out of control. But Jarred kept saying I felt so good, so warm,
so soft that I put my fears aside and let myself go. Then I came,
milk started spurting from my breasts, and the baby woke up and
started crying like it somehow got the signal. I brought it into bed
to nurse while Jarred licked milk from my other nipple—not ex-
actly what I'd expected, but pretty satisfying all in all.

Leaking milk, by the way, is normal with orgasm because of let-down stimulated by oxytocin. As for the baby waking at the exact moment of orgasm, it's been noted that prolactin tends to synchronize mother–infant sleep cycles, causing a kind of physiological empathy between the two.

This brings us to yet another area of concern, that of sleeping arrangements for the baby. In the last few decades, family sleeping—baby or children in bed with their parents—has seen a surge of popularity in the United States. Reports from those who have tried it are generally positive. At least in the beginning, having the baby in bed makes a big difference in how much sleep the mother gets: Often, she is able to nurse without fully awakening. The risk of rolling on top of the baby has proven to be just a myth, and increased skin-to-skin intimacy has emotional benefits for both parents and child. However, if it gets to the point where you and your partner are sleeping in separate beds, it's time to reconsider the arrangement.

A wise pediatrician friend suggests that right from the start, parents put the baby on its own little mattress (or in a bassinet) next to their bed, at least for part of the night. This may help the baby get used to sleeping alone, if only part time. One mother relayed that after a particularly difficult night, she and her partner decided to move their ten-month-old daughter to another room, and she suddenly began sleeping through the night; apparently she had been disturbed by her parents' noises. But the mother also noted that this was not a permanent arrangement; in a few weeks, her daughter was back sleeping with them again. Sleeping all night in solitude is uncommon for little ones, and they may climb into their parents' bed in the wee hours of the morning for many years to come.

How does this work in terms of sex? It depends on the age of the child; if yours is still an infant and you find yourself interrupted in the middle of something sweet, you may decide to quietly continue. Many women report the stopgap solution of nursing the baby while making love: an odd juggle of emotions, but eminently practical.

Your toddler will probably be a bit too aware for this sort of thing. Still, be sure to let your little one see you and your partner cozily hugging and kissing, lest this behavior lead to anxiety should she or he come upon you unawares. Of course, any child will be less jealous and possessive if regularly given lots of love and affection.

Ultimately, new parents make do. And they become creative, seeking out different times and places for an intimate rendezvous. See the forthcoming section, "Recapturing Intimacy," for further suggestions.

Sexual Difficulties

◎

Sometimes, more than the usual emotional adjustments or practical concerns affect postpartum sexuality. Any serious setback in physical recuperation, or a traumatic event like the death of a loved one, loss of a job, or a sudden need to relocate can have a major effect on libido.

If it has not already surfaced, deep-seated ambivalence about gender roles may arise in the father. If he is harboring the Madonna/Whore dichotomy, this may be the breaking point. Perhaps he was able to love his partner during the pregnancy, but now finds himself deeply uncomfortable relating to her as a mother. She may notice that he seems hesitant to touch her and think it's because her looks have changed or that she is no longer sexually enticing, while the real reason is his own internal conflict. Some men respond by having affairs; others plunge into their work or some recreational activity. Either way, home life suffers, and intervention is called for. Bear in mind that the postpartum period may be the first (and perhaps the most critical) time for a man to face up to misogynist attitudes at odds with his better judgment. There is nothing easy about this process, but it can lead in the long run to more intimate ways of living and loving.

For herself, a woman may feel frustrated and conflicted in the roles of mother, lover, and career woman. As long as she reassures her partner that these conflicts have nothing whatsoever to do with his or her adequacy, they will have a chance at intimacy. She may find, however, that she must set new boundaries in the relationship: something of a taboo for women in this culture but essential nonetheless. New mothers need to conserve their energy, and a major way to do this is to say no to anything that conflicts with their instincts. Setting boundaries means being honest, not holding back. Key phrases include: "I can't____. Could you____?"; "No, not right now"; "Can we talk about it later?"; and finally, "I need to get some rest."

In the same vein, it is important to be realistic about sex in this phase. The combination of bone-weary fatigue, interruptions from the baby, and/or worry about finances, household matters, and work schedules is hardly conducive to joyous and spontaneous lovemaking. This simply is not one of those honeymoon times when sex is a breeze. This needn't cause panic, though, if both partners keep things in perspective by realizing that this phase is only temporary. This is really what intimate partnership is all about— keeping the long view, and loving as much as we can along the way.

Sylvia reports:

I felt very estranged from my body and so tired all the time I didn't want sex at all. But Mark would put pressure on me. Then I'd get in the mood, and he'd be too worn out, worried or something. Finally, I got in the habit of shutting him out, until one day he broke down and told me how much he missed me, missed our closeness. Really, I had forgotten that he cared, that I cared. The birth just turned me upside down, I guess, and I was so involved with the baby.

I told him what it was like for me, how exhausted and used up I felt, and as we talked, one thing led to another and we were making love. It sure wasn't perfect (the baby actually interrupted with a nursing) but it was real. You know that quality, when sex is ultra-real? It was raw, it was different, it was new—we were three now, instead of two, more instead of less. Once I saw this, staying connected to Mark became easier. We got really good at blending sex into ordinary, day-to-day things we did, so that when we were alone, we got intimate right away. I felt like I had discovered the secret to a happy marriage and wondered, "How come no one ever told me about this?"

When we learn to support each other in spite of stress, or even because of it, our sexual experience takes on more meaning. When we make love in order to learn and grow, setting aside expectations and taking from sex whatever we find, we have entered a new stage of sexual maturity. The challenges of the postpartum period initiate this evolution.

Recapturing Intimacy

◎

Ideally, intimacy is not seriously interrupted or lost in the process of giving birth. But there is change, as discussed, and sometimes a couple must work to reestablish closeness and trust. This means talking about sex, communicating hurts, fears, and desires more openly than ever before. With a baby around, it also means making an effort to be emotionally and sexually available to each other, even when one partner is not fully in the mood. It means picking up where you left off, even though days may intervene, by keeping your intimacy alive in heart and deed.

Remember that you cannot have deep intimacy in relationship unless you find time to be intimate with yourself. Time alone is *not* a luxury—it is a necessity! You do not have to have a hot date with your partner or some important business matter to justify hiring a babysitter or asking a friend or relative to watch the baby for a few hours. Use this time for yourself lovingly: relax, be aware of your feelings, do something pleasurable or inspiring, be in touch with your soul's purpose.

Here are a few well-seasoned tips for keeping the fires burning:

1. **Have some ritual in your sex life.** Choose a night once a week to have dinner and watch a video after the baby is asleep, and then have sex right there on the floor, on the couch, in the spare bedroom, or wherever takes your fancy. Even if you are interrupted and can't resume, you know your next special evening is only a week away.

2. **Get out.** Find a good babysitter willing to commit to a certain night each week. Choose someone you know and trust or seek recommendations from those closest to you. Going out regularly makes a difference: The benefits build up. Once out, you may talk mostly about the baby, but try to talk about yourselves, too.

3. **Make cooking and housework as easy as possible.** If you ever planned to treat yourself to hired help, now is the time to do it. If this is not affordable, buy a slow cooker for meals that practically cook themselves, or resort to the microwave. I also tell my clients to farm out dinner preparation for the first two weeks postpartum by enlisting every friend or relative who offers assistance or wants to come see the baby. You

can also cook casseroles and soups in advance and freeze as much as possible.

4. **Insist on time alone.** This is time for your spirit, time you make sacred by having fun, renewing yourself, making sure you are well from the inside out. Start doing this now, and don't ever stop! And don't let anyone interrupt you or make you feel guilty about taking this much-needed time for yourself.

5. **Develop a sense of humor.** If you don't have one already, you will definitely need it in the years ahead. Let your troubles roll off your shoulders. Joke around with your partner, your kids, and yourself. Call good friends for a chat and some silliness. Let your heart be light, and look on the bright side of difficult situations.

6. **Try not to burden your partner with grim realities, at least not on the emotional level.** If you can translate your troubles into specific needs and instructions, okay, but otherwise, forget it. Take responsibility for what you feel. Try to find your own ways of alleviating stress and making yourself feel better. Find others to talk to for solace and inspiration.

7. **Know that this wild and crazy time will pass.** Maintain the long view, plan your first weekend (or weeklong) getaway with pleasure, and keep the faith.

Against all odds, many women feel their sexuality to be greatly enhanced by giving birth. Some have orgasms for the first time in their lives. Perhaps this is because birth partners a woman with herself: The keys to letting go and making progress in labor come from within her. Especially if she has been buffeted around by male needs, desires, and opinions about sex, birth can be quite a revelation. As Cassie says:

I never had orgasms like I did after giving birth. When I was pushing my daughter out, I was more than connected to my vaginal muscles—I actually became them. My strength was incredible, my timing exquisite. Before, when I made love it was me up here, vagina down there. But now my awareness and intelligence are fully inside me. I'm not afraid to do or try anything with my body; its power belongs to me. Once you've let go giving birth, letting go with sex can take you to places you've never dreamed of.

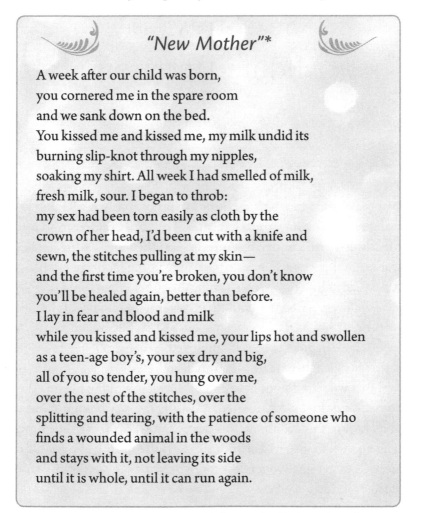

"New Mother"*

A week after our child was born,
you cornered me in the spare room
and we sank down on the bed.
You kissed me and kissed me, my milk undid its
burning slip-knot through my nipples,
soaking my shirt. All week I had smelled of milk,
fresh milk, sour. I began to throb:
my sex had been torn easily as cloth by the
crown of her head, I'd been cut with a knife and
sewn, the stitches pulling at my skin—
and the first time you're broken, you don't know
you'll be healed again, better than before.
I lay in fear and blood and milk
while you kissed and kissed me, your lips hot and swollen
as a teen-age boy's, your sex dry and big,
all of you so tender, you hung over me,
over the nest of the stitches, over the
splitting and tearing, with the patience of someone who
finds a wounded animal in the woods
and stays with it, not leaving its side
until it is whole, until it can run again.

* From *The Dead and the Living* by Sharon Olds (New York: Alfred Knopf, 1984).

◎

CHAPTER 6

Sex, Stress, *and* *the* Midlife Turnaround

Women of today are beyond busy. We precariously juggle the demands of work, our primary relationships, our children, and our friendships with our personal needs. And then there is the housework: running errands, paying bills, purchasing food and clothing, supervising household repairs, doing the cooking and laundry. If we have children, we confer with their teachers and help with homework on a regular basis. With luck, once in a while we lunch with a friend. If we happen to be self-employed, or are struggling to make career advances, we are definitely in deep water!

Most women do not have a choice about working outside the home. Even if we are partnered, it usually takes two wage earners to make it in this economy. This has been true for some time now, long enough to give us a chance to assess the quality of our hectic lifestyle. Increasingly, our needs for rejuvenation are swept aside for greater productivity. Few of us practice genuine rituals of self-care. We are lucky to be at work on time, survive the day's annoyances, handle personal business, and get dinner on the table. Later, we collapse into bed with little energy to talk or touch. Most of us barely get by each day, let alone find time for pleasure and intimacy.

Is there no way out of this dilemma? Before we can realistically discuss the effect of the superwoman syndrome on sexuality, we must realize how incompatible the two really are. In so many ways, lack of time for self-care negates sexual desire.

Of course, there are stopgap measures like the weekend getaway, lunch-break rendezvous, or quiet evening in. These do help to maintain a sense of balance by providing relief from tension. But ultimately, snatched moments together are not enough, because real intimacy cannot be staged or forced; it must be based on genuine and deep communication. If communication is continually fragmented, disrupted, or shelved indefinitely, sudden episodes of private time can end up in arguments or long, involved discussions that sap rather than renew us. As Margaret reported:

> *We'd start out with a romantic meal or something, then wild and crazy sex. But when we finally got down to talking later, all that emerged was frustration and resentment. I just don't get it—why do I have to do it all? The daily routine is bad enough, but even when I'm supposedly free, I'm initiating talks and fielding the upsets. I feel unseen, invisible. I'm taking care of everything and everybody, but nobody cares for me.*

Transforming Gender-Based Expectations

◎

Margaret's lament hits it right on the mark for many of us. Unfortunately, the solution isn't any easier to bear than the problem, but here it is: The only one who can really take care of Margaret is Margaret herself. She must revamp her priorities so that her own are at the top. Further, her entire gender role must be recast from serving others to nurturing herself. This is a drastic shift from what many of our mothers believed and what society continues to expect of us.

This is especially difficult in a society that refuses to accord women equal rights and privileges to those of men. Men as a group have a higher pay scale, greater social security benefits, more free time, and more opportunity to play than women. With our role as servant so deeply entrenched in our social structure, in the institutions of marriage, education, health care, business, and religion, we are going to have to assert loud and clear just exactly what we need, and how and when we need it. As Camille Paglia says, "Feminism begins at home. It begins with every single woman drawing the line."[1] At first, this seems like just another job to do. But this is a worthwhile task, one that can cause inappropriate or demeaning roles to fall by the wayside. The need to assert ourselves is more than a personal issue; it is a political, social, and ecological imperative.

Here is a quote from Sedonia Cahill, contributor to *The Women's Wheel of Life*:

It is nearly impossible not to get stuck in mothering in our society. That's certainly the role that the culture prefers, as far as I can tell. Women's basic and very good impulse to mother children has been so exploited by the patriarchy that they end up being mother to grown men, who are free to behave like children and become very boring. It's a major cause of dissension between men and women, this exploitation—there's such a pull to keep us locked into that place.

To break out of being defined as a nurturer, a woman has to commit to her own life, and doing that is scary—choosing yourself instead of someone else is really a frightening thing to do, like you're being a bad girl. But even as a mother, you have to make a commitment to your own life. And I don't think that can be done without a circle of sisters, where you learn to feel good and wonderful about yourself, see yourself reflected in the eyes of women that you love very much—it helps you decide you are worth it, that your own life really must come first."[2]

For years, women have been taught to be the peacemakers, to soothe and field the emotional problems of others to the exclusion of their own. When we behave this way with men, it's no wonder that we find them out of touch with their feelings. It is true that men have biological difficulties, due to brain structure and function, in linking emotion to other aspects of behavior and response. But why should we go so far as to translate their emotions for them? Perhaps we would find less resentment on their part if we focused our efforts on putting our feelings, needs, and desires forward overtly, rather than covertly. This is a different model of relationship than what most of us have imprinted, but it could serve to create a healthier sort of intimacy.

One woman shared these words from her husband: "You know, you women think you have it so hard, but at least you know what you're fighting for. You've got principles—for us guys, if we start to open up and change, it's pretty confusing." Although we may feel compassion for men in this quandary, we must continuously beware of any tendency to rescue them. When we do, we perpetuate the problem by colluding with it.

Women have been accused of being angry and reactive, but so are men. Our anger is easy to root in inequality, overwork, and unsupportive social structures: In short, we are angry at society. For men, society is basically supportive and therefore not the target, but women frequently are. Rape is obvious evidence of this; violent pornography further serves to illustrate. Men are angry with women for brushing them off, abandoning them to their own confusion, failing to make the pain and frustration of life easier to bear. And it's true that many of us are just too busy to bother with male angst as we once did.

On the other hand, the stress of competing in a man's world has led some women to adopt male characteristics almost to the exclusion of their own. So deeply have we rebelled against being stereotyped as weak, indecisive, and irrational that some of us have inadvertently rejected the positive side of these aspects: sensitivity, flexibility, and the creativity to discern and chart our own course. True, we may have been forced to do this to advance in our careers. But perhaps the time has come to reincorporate these feminine aspects into our way of life, our approach to problem solving, and our intimate relationships.

In his book *Men, Women and Relationships*, John Gray describes four patterns commonly found in intimate partnerships. Of particular relevance to this discussion is the pattern in which a woman is reactively independent, so much so that she severs critical ties with herself and others. We know her by the following: (1) she is overly defensive; (2) she is compulsively organized and responsible; (3) she is suspicious, cold, and critical; (4) she is pushy and manipulative; (5) she is tense, intolerant, judgmental, and impatient; and (6) she is unable to accept support.[3] Not surprisingly, she tends to choose a partner who is weak, dependent, and unfocused. It is easy to see how many of the brightest and most creative women of our time have ended up this way. But this unnatural, constricted state of being is clearly at odds with a woman's chances for health and happiness, sexual pleasure and intimacy.

As Stacy relates:

I kept blaming Bob, but I knew it was me. I had become so sharp with him, so on edge all the time, so critical and controlling, that we just didn't get along. I convinced myself that sex was still fine; after all, I knew exactly how to let my guard down in bed. But the chemistry between us, the erotic side of our day-to-day contact, was missing.

Like women who have repressed their feminine traits, men who subdue their masculine traits may find themselves less dynamic in their relationships or life in general. Yes, it is good for men to be open, sensitive, and easygoing at times, but chronic indecisiveness or irresponsibility are signs of trouble. Particularly when a man begins to live on dreams, or becomes moody and withdrawn much of the time, something is definitely wrong.

With male and female aspects out of balance, sex will invariably be affected because the fundamental attraction between opposites has been disrupted. The most common mistake in relationships is trying to make our partner more like we are, more manageable and predictable. As our differences diminish, so will the attraction. We turn into friends instead of lovers: The passion is gone. Gray states, "To whatever extent a partner must suppress their ways of being, feeling, thinking, or doing in order to receive love or be safe in a relationship, the passion will fade."

Perhaps this accounts in part for the great popularity of E. L. James' *Fifty Shades of Gray* trilogy. Jokingly dubbed "mommy porn," its theme of sadomasochism touched a nerve in our culture, that of the repression and frustration all too common in long-term relationships. That it also speaks vividly to the impacts of abuse on sexuality is, sadly, another major factor in its widespread appeal.

Repression of self and other is a complex matter and not easy to remedy. One approach is to acknowledge and engage both our feminine and masculine traits, while keeping an eye on the balance. As mentioned above, some women need to deliberately evoke the feminine, which may be facilitated by seeking the company of other women for discussion and processing. Changes in lifestyle, in the daily blend of activity and rest, may also be called for, and sometimes the only way to accomplish this is by breaking routine or taking a vacation.

In any event, women need intimate relationships in life. Close, healthy ties with others help us reconnect with ourselves. Remember that women generally solve problems by talking matters through with friends or family, formulating and evolving their thoughts aloud. This propensity to share "half-baked truths," in contrast to men's preference for airing already polished positions, has been referred to by women themselves as "real talk."[4] It is time we acknowledge that certain needs readily met by women are rarely satisfied by men.

Let us return to the importance of circling for women. As women move through their thirties, they begin to recognize the power of menstruation and to truly appreciate their monthly rounds of moods and aptitudes. Most settle into a regular rhythm, and many find synchronous cycling with female coworkers or housemates to be fairly consistent. As they approach their forties, they may begin to celebrate these joint moon times, using them for deep discussion and renewal. This process of biological alignment is known as entrainment. Menstrual entrainment is the basis for what I term "blood bonding," that is, the deep interconnectedness of women who intentionally share their menstrual wisdom and vision to unite. Blood bonding takes women's circling up a notch; it makes possible a level of work and play heretofore unknown to younger women.

What does this have to do with revamping gender-based expectations? The stronger women are in their own ways of knowing and being, the less inclined they are to fuss and worry about their differences with men. If asked, most men wish women would speak to them calmly, giving them clear and simple instructions rather than process or diatribe. This is an important indication of why women need to circle, and how circling can, albeit indirectly, improve their relationships with men.

Nevertheless, shifts in gender-based expectations carry the liability of loss, whether of identity in the relationship, familiar patterns of interaction, or sexual intimacy. These losses are usually temporary, but they can be worrisome.

Susan reveals:

When I started to be truthful with my partner about what I needed, I was pretty scared. Scared he wouldn't love me, wouldn't care, or even worse, couldn't help me. We were both surprised, I think, to find that our relationship actually endured, and things began to change for the better. But for a while, we couldn't make love. A lot was being stirred up for both of us.

If estrangement persists in a relationship, the underlying issues must be identified. A couple might be able to manage this on their own, or they may need the help of a professional. In any event, when dealing with shifts in gender roles, a little patience goes a long way—it can give both parties a chance to stretch, experiment, grow, and reach new depths of understanding essential for any long-term solution.

Sex and Anger
◎

On the other hand, if there is deep-seated anger in a relationship, sexual intimacy will all but vanish. As expert Marilyn Ruman, PhD, says, "Anger is almost always the enemy of desire and is one of the best places to look when your sex life is floundering."[5]

Unfortunately, anger is often repressed or unconscious in relationships. Typically, the angry partner will try to force the other to act it out, while taking a turn at resistance and avoidance. These patterns usually have roots in a childhood with parents doing much the same, enacting extremes of submission and domination. Particularly when chemical dependency, physical abuse, or sexual abuse are part of the family history, a survivor comes to believe (and rightly so, in such situations) that expressing anger is dangerous and will lead to unhappiness.

An unhealthy relationship to anger is endemic of patriarchy, with its hierarchical structure of privilege based on "power over" rather than "power with" others. In truth, anger is a normal emotion, nothing to feel ashamed of. It's what we do with it that counts. If we enact patriarchal values by using our anger to try to control others, we miss its real purpose in our lives, which is to spur us to take a stand against injustice, cruelty, and violence.

The shadow side of anger is sadness and loss. If there are unresolved traumas in the family history that have filtered into the relationship, these must be worked through before there can be any hope of intimacy. Time is of the essence, though, especially for the relationship in which anger has been repressed but is now beginning to explode. The longer a couple has been holding back and accumulating resentment, the more each will expect—or may try to force—the other to make it up to them. This can lead to various forms of abuse, and also illustrates why patterns of dependency and abuse tend to be self-perpetuating.

One way to work with anger is to recognize that it correlates to need. It is important to acknowledge our anger, yes, but it is even more critical to articulate the need it represents. If a couple can agree to deal with anger as it arises by making time to hear each other's needs, and attempting either to meet them or negotiate alternatives, intimacy may soon resurface.

It may also be necessary to weed out patterns of avoidance in the relationship. Spending inordinate amounts of time in separate parts of the house, taking meals separately, going to bed at different times, or arguing just before bed are classic examples of repressed anger, as are not taking care of oneself physically, neglecting shared environments (particularly the bedroom), or cluttering free time with small talk and busywork. Deliberate changes in these areas can prompt discussion, but should this escalate to confrontation that only makes matters worse, professional help is called for.

Stress and Sexuality

◎

Stress, too, is an enemy of desire. Consider the physical effects of stress, particularly on the adrenal glands. The adrenals have two parts, the medulla and the cortex. When we are stressed, the medulla produces catecholamines, one of which is adrenaline, responsible for our flight-or-fight response when threatened or in danger. The cortex is responsible for producing the sex hormones estrogen and progesterone, but more significantly, the testosterone responsible for libido. To some degree, these functions are opposing; for example, if stress is chronic or protracted so that the medulla must continually pump the body with catecholamines, androgen production from the cortex may be neglected. Here we have a physiological explanation of how stress may dampen sexual desire.

Psychologically, stress causes us to either fight or withdraw. Sexual activity under these circumstances simply may not occur, or it may be brief and explosive. Nothing wrong with the latter, except that it precludes the comfort and intimacy essential in any long-term relationship. The situation is even more difficult if both partners are under stress. The challenges of trying to unwind in bed, encountering emotions carefully held in check while trying to coordinate with another doing the same, can be uncomfortable enough to dissuade both from making the effort.

Some couples manage nonsexual phases by keeping the communication going in other ways, particularly through shared activities that both enjoy. Others choose to have sex—whether good, bad, or indifferent—to maintain some degree of connection. Either way, couples suffering from chronic stress will find it an obstacle to intimacy. The answer lies not in the bedroom, but in coming to terms with the problem and responding to it intelligently. From Natalie:

> *It's rough for us right now: We both knock ourselves out at work, the kids get little of our attention, we both feel guilty and angry, and we often take it out on each other. Then we have sex to make up. Sometimes it's great, a real release. Sometimes it just doesn't make it; we're still all bottled up, and we feel more separate than before. But that's marriage, I guess.*

To complicate matters, men and women generally have different reactions to stress. Whereas men tend to withdraw to consider the situation, women respond with a rush of emotion, wanting more than anything else to sift through their feelings and discuss them to find some stability. For most women, this is the only way they can separate their needs from the needs of others and avoid becoming overwhelmed.

Women who are overwhelmed have one characteristic in common: They lose the ability to prioritize.[6] Every task and obligation suddenly assumes equal importance. Whether it's finishing up a project on a deadline or loading the dishwasher, everything is done in a continuous overwrought stream of activity, rather like a runaway train.

The more we become overwhelmed, the more likely we are to overreact to the inconsequential. Not being able to distinguish the important issues, we focus our frustration and anger on little irritations. Every woman knows the idiotic feeling of exploding in fury over the unwashed dish in the sink, or the single paper napkin scuttling about the floor. At this point, total exhaustion is forthcoming: We feel utterly drained, useless, and alone. This scenario takes its toll on everyone who loves us.

When we hit bottom, we see clearly that the long-suffering, self-negating approach to stress and its causes does not work. Unfortunately, we often forget this lesson as we reemerge from the depths; we try to normalize quickly, put on a happy face, and get back to work, only to have the pattern repeat again. This is because our culture teaches us to fear the depths, to equate the experience of falling apart and hitting bottom with psychosis or depression. When we go deep into the well of being, we cease to be available to others and are no longer "productive." Yet this process, known as *descent* in numerous spiritual traditions, is really a sacred one.

Descent gives us the opportunity to rest at the core of our existence. If we fully surrender, we may experience great insight and rejuvenation that stays with us. But if we fight descent or try to reemerge from it before we are ready, we miss the point and are apt to be plagued with anxiety or bouts of true depression.

Here is a quote from Adele Getty, contributor to *The Women's Wheel of Life*:

> *The image I had of myself was of being on a large, black sea, madly flailing around like a many-armed goddess, every arm flailing on the surface of the water as I tried to stay afloat. Finally, in the midst of this panic I called for help and said, "What is this about*

and what can I do? This is taking a lot of energy, trying to stay afloat." I couldn't sleep, and no matter what I tried to do during the day, psychically I was flailing. And this voice just came and said, "Surrender, just drown, just let go and drown." I stopped flailing and I let myself drown—and I drowned, but I didn't die. I sank into this sea of peace, calmness, serenity…no, serenity is too strong…it didn't have the positive energy serenity has, but there was nothing negative about it. It was emptiness, and it wasn't taking any energy anymore and it was all right, I could just be there in this emptiness. It wasn't blissful but I could sleep, and immediately the energetics of my life shifted and started supporting me again. But if I tried to jump in with both feet, pick up the ball and run with it, I immediately got smashed back down. A month would go by and I'd think, "Surely I can start being actively engaged in this process," but nope, I'd be wrong…and this went on for nine months. My natural tendency is to bob back up and start running, but my challenge was not to emerge too soon from the underworld. Making the descent is a process, being in the underworld is a process, and making the ascent, slowly coming back is a process too, and if you short circuit any step along the way, you're going to have to go though the journey again.[7]

On the other hand, if stress is chronic due to addiction, unemployment, illness, or other crises involving a loved one or family member, outside help is essential. There may be no immediate solution, but at least the difficulty can be tempered with support. When in high-stress situations like these, we must continue to care for and nurture ourselves, as this is the only way we can possibly meet the challenges of caring for others. Beyond support, we need our own outside activities, some structure and routine, meaningful work to do. Sex may be low on the list of priorities when we are in dire straits: Certainly this makes sense physiologically. Or, with intention, it may serve as the glue that keeps us together.

How Children Affect Sexuality

◎

For those who have children, let's look at how family life can influence sexuality. We will begin with an overview of the key developmental phases in children's lives and how these might affect a woman's inclination for and enjoyment of sex.

T. Berry Brazelton, authority on child rearing and development, observes that when a child reaches the age of two, the parents may begin to compete for his or her affections.[8] Why does this occur? Considering how little time parents of a toddler have for themselves and each other, they can easily become sexually estranged. And then, for want of privacy and intimacy, they may transfer their needs onto their child and vie bitterly for his or her attention.

If this situation is left unaddressed, studies show that the likelihood of extramarital affairs is high, reaching a peak when the child is three or four. Once the couple is past this critical point, the survival issues of the first few years have been surmounted—and parents have an opportunity to view the wreckage. If there is ever a time when parents need and deserve a vacation, it is now.

Here are some practical suggestions that might help to forestall such a crisis.

Take Private Time

Again, this is not optional! It is the *only* way to find the energy to relate intimately with your partner. Try to squeeze a bit of time out of your usual routine. Simplify meals so you have free time before dinner. Do household chores in chunks, running several tasks simultaneously to save time and steps. Lower your standards for neatness and cleanliness.

A more lasting approach is to change your routines so that time for yourself is built in. Right from the start, teach your children ways to take care of themselves. Those of us whose parents struggled to give us the best of everything may need to unlearn certain self-sacrificing behaviors. In a healthy family, every member does his or her share. If you are in a position to hire additional help, do it. Save your relationship by taking care of yourself first and foremost.

Sociologist Pepper Schwartz of the University of Washington identifies three types of marriage arrangements: (1) traditional marriage; (2) near-peer marriage; and (3) peer marriage. Traditional unions are those wherein partners play conventional gender roles, with sharply divided tasks and responsibilities. In near-peer unions, both have jobs, but one still does the majority of housework and child rearing. Peer unions are fully egalitarian matches: Each partner has equal rank and is responsible for both the economic and emotional well-being of the household, with chores divided equally. As you might expect, those in peer unions report an intense sense of companionship and high levels of intimacy.[9]

Housework is such a charged issue for most couples that it deserves a few more words. As for keys to an enduring marriage, author Andrew Ward dryly advises, "It doesn't matter if one of you spends all day on the patio eating bonbons, you've got to divide housework right down the middle. Actual equalized work schedules, impervious to the shirker and martyr among you (shirkers and martyrs compose most married couples), should be hammered out right away and signed, preferably in blood, by both parties."[10]

Keep Up With Your Dreams

Don't let your dreams fade so that you no longer remember them. Take time to review your long-term goals and fantasies of what could be, giving yourself the freedom to be visionary. Where do you want to be a year from now, or five, or ten years hence? What must you absolutely do in life to feel you have really lived? Some say that whatever you loved to do most when aged seven or eight holds a key to your future. Think back, dream forward, and keep track of what you see.

Make Time for the Relationship

When you are busy, intimacy must be made a priority. This means creating "couple time," literally scheduling it in. Maintain a weekly date night. And choose another time, perhaps in the morning when you are both fresh, to talk about what is going on in your lives and how you are feeling. This time of open disclosure works best if you both agree to hear each other out without interrupting or being judgmental. Some couples do this daily, others once a week: The more you practice this, the more it will occur spontaneously.

Never underestimate the power of an entire night alone together. There is a dramatic difference between sex when you know you might be interrupted and sex with total privacy. Plus, it's nice to have the freedom to resume again later in the evening if you feel like it. At least twice a year, make plans to get away to some romantic location. When you are embroiled in family life, you must work to re-create your love.

Surprise Yourself and Your Lover

Do the unexpected once in a while. When your love was young, it was exciting to try new things together, share adventures, and discover your commonalities in a variety of situations. Let this element of excitement back into your life, and don't worry about appearing foolish. Take a few risks on new activities, and update your style to reflect your growth. Often, we marry (or make long-term commitments) because we want stability: We want a nice, simple routine. But routine is routine—it needs the spice of innovation to keep it from becoming dull. Reanimate yourself with new experiences, new impressions. This is a time-honored way of stimulating creativity and passion.

Get Help If You Need It

Marriage or couple counseling doesn't have to be a long-term proposition. People often end up in counseling because it is the only way they seem able to make the time to talk to one another. The main benefit of counseling is that it provides an opportunity to be witnessed. Someone who is objective about your problems can re-frame them in ways that make it easier for you to handle them on your own. Almost every intimate partnership needs a boost like this once in a while.

◎   ◎   ◎

A critical period for mothers is that when their child begins school full-time. The child is no longer fully dependent, and all the trap-pings of that phase come to an end. The mother who has been free to stay at home will suddenly have lots of time during the day—so much that she may be at a loss for ways to fill it. On the other hand, the mother who has been unable to spend much time with her child may feel longing for the irreplaceable phase she has missed. These emotions may be difficult to explain to one's partner because they are closely linked to the mother–infant bond—though increasingly, male (or female) partners who provide close care in the early years have these feelings too. But those not so intimately involved tend to dismiss these empty-nest blues as the height of irrationality. They remember the sleepless nights, the mad shuffle for babysitters, the interrupted lovemaking, and above all, their partner's complaints, and wonder how she can possibly be serious.

Then again, over the years a number of my clients have con-fessed that they really didn't want to be mothers and so experience great relief at this point. Making peace with your truth as a mother is essential to your mental and sexual health—if this is you, don't compare yourself to those who love mothering and are very happy in that role. That the media has interpreted these differences in at-titude and the parenting styles they represent as "Mommy Wars" is just another example of cultural exploitation of the superwoman concept (to be discussed in the next section).

Still, at this juncture, most mothers must reestablish their iden-tity and set new goals for themselves and their primary relationship.

Now is the time to recall pre-motherhood ambitions that remain unfulfilled. Particularly if a woman has given up her career for motherhood and is thinking of going back to work, she must take a hard look at how far she has fallen behind.

In any period of change, we use what we have been as a springboard for what we wish to become. Listen to what Christine has to say:

> *I was happy Zoe was off to school, but I did feel a little empty. Especially with my husband—I just couldn't make him understand. Really, I didn't understand it myself, until one day it was suddenly clear. Before, when I was recovering from the birth and trying to get my body back, I wanted him to love me for what I was before— to remind me, you know? Now, with Zoe out in the world, I want him to reaffirm me for the mother I have become, and let me know I don't have to be anything else.*

Again, we have an example of a woman wanting reassurance from her partner that she really needs to give to herself. It is important that we search our feelings for the seeds of our own direction, and respond accordingly.

From ages five to seven, children identify with the family unit; thereafter they begin to relate to society at large. And then comes adolescence. Many mothers find their adolescent daughters to be particularly challenging. I recall describing mine at age eleven as being in "a perpetual state of PMS." This is the time when girls become extremely critical of their mothers, particularly as regards personal appearance. I remember coming down the stairs dressed for a party one night when my daughter remarked most caustically, "You're not going to wear *that*, are you?" The stress is compounded if Mom has reached a major chronological landmark of her own—say, her fortieth birthday. In spite of herself, she may end up making expensive trips to the cosmetics counter, beauty salon, or dieters group. Not that this is necessarily bad, but the upshot may be persisting uncertainty about her physical attractiveness.

The natural shift in power that occurs in adolescence may further complicate matters. Especially if your parenting style has been to press your will on your young ones, their natural rebellion at this age can leave you feeling powerless. And in truth, the role of parent does begin to shift from director to guide and confidant. If (for whatever reason) you too are in upheaval, this change in your role may feel like yet another blow to your self-confidence. Counseling or professional help is a good idea, as this is no time to be reactive or forceful with your children.

The "bread baking" approach to child rearing goes like this: You mix and add ingredients when children are young, you watch the dough rise (and must deflate it occasionally) as they mature, but once the bread is in the oven of adolescence, you had best not open the door! Sure, you keep an eye on things, but you don't interfere unless the bread is about to burn.

The Midlife Turnaround

◎

Superwomen and supermoms come in all ages. But depending on the decade of a woman's life, she will have particular sexual needs and orientation. Sex in young adulthood is largely about identifying with and pleasing another as a means of self-discovery. Sex in the thirties tends to focus on pair bonding and procreation. Sex in midlife reestablishes the priorities of the self: physical, emotional, and spiritual. Taking the long view, it makes sense that the big push for security and success during our twenties and thirties might lead to a values and identity crisis in our forties. It should come as no surprise that a similar crisis might follow sexually.

Our cultural image of midlife crisis is that of older man, younger woman. This, from Barbara, illustrates how a woman in midlife can find meaning in weathering such an experience:

My husband had affairs from the time he turned forty, and I only found out three years later. I was so furious, so humiliated that I really didn't think we were going to make it. Couldn't sleep with him at all, but he wanted to stay, so we had counseling. All that stuff, I'll spare you—but when we finally started making love again, I was a different woman. I went out for myself. Whenever the pain of his betrayal would start to get to me, I'd hold on to myself and just do what I felt was best for me. I got in touch with a strength I didn't know I had, and I aligned myself with it, even in bed.

Of course, many women choose to cut their losses on pain like this and move on. Some have affairs of their own, in search of healing. Others become obsessed with their attractiveness, doing anything to stay young. But what Barbara referred to as aligning with her strength is increasingly crucial, as it enables us to meet challenges to our health and identity as we continue to age. Is it not therefore fitting that in midlife, we should seek to explore and express ourselves as never before? "Forty and fabulous": We know what we like, we speak our minds, we have a solid base from which to innovate, and pleasure is ours for the taking!

Here's an interesting comment from a friend a few weeks after her fortieth birthday:

I thought midlife crises were only for men. But it's really hit me...I'm turning into a real loudmouth, saying things to my boss and husband I wouldn't have dreamed of saying before! You figure you have only so much time...I feel almost ruthless about getting my needs met.

And what was this doing to her sex life?

This is pretty personal, but in the middle of making love one night I just blurted out, "Joe, why don't you concentrate?" I never said anything like that before...see, my husband just tends to ramble on sometimes in bed, without focusing on me. When he paused (I guess he was a little shocked), I added, "You know, concentrate on me." I couldn't believe I did that!

It is a well-known fact that men reach their sexual peak (as per intensity and endurance) in their early twenties, but women reach theirs later, often in the forties. This is partly physical, partly psychological. For many women, it takes that long to get to know themselves sexually, to overcome taboos of sexual self-expression, to trust their bodies and be confident enough to get what they want in bed.

This is also a time when women who have never fantasized before find their sexual imagination coming to life. In her book *Women on Top*, Nancy Friday explores the range and outrageousness of women's fantasies as they reach this peak. Interestingly, these fantasies tend to be physically oriented, focused on ways of maximizing sensation, while the fantasies of younger women are more emotionally based. For example, a woman in her twenties might fantasize about a long romantic buildup and the preludes to lovemaking, whereas the midlife woman will focus more on sexual positions and her partner's techniques, or even on bondage and multiple partners as enhancements to her sensation.

June Reinisch, in *The Kinsey Report*, notes that men and women do a turnaround in sexual temperament at this point. As women become more intrigued with physical experimentation, men become interested in letting themselves be vulnerable and caring.[11] These changes are hormonally based, for as women approach menopause, their reproductive hormones surge intensely to force ovulation. Thus women tracking their cycles commonly report fertile peaks like never before, with ovulation so intense that, as one woman put it, "I'm wet to my knees with fertile mucus!" Testosterone levels also rise dramatically in the forties. But for men of the same age, testosterone begins to decrease. In effect, women become more masculine, and men, more feminine. This explains a little-appreciated fact about men in midlife crisis: If they seek younger women, it is not so much for the wild reenactment of youthful passion but because these women are sexually oriented precisely as they themselves wish to be, emotionally and romantically. This strikes women in their forties as the height of irony—all those years they yearned for romance, while he wanted nothing but sex! Thus some women at this age form liaisons with younger men, but changing the sexual dynamics in an established partnership can also make the most of these facts of life.

Testosterone levels do, in fact, correlate to the degree of aggressiveness in women and, in many cases, to a disinclination to stay in monogamous relationships. A study conducted by Patricia Schreiner-Engel, associate professor of obstetrics/gynecology and psychiatry at Mount Sinai School of Medicine in New York, found that women in the most powerful career positions had the highest testosterone levels, and few were in long-term relationships. On the other hand, women with lower testosterone levels were often homemakers, students, or temporary workers, and they tended to have enduring marriages.

Socioeconomic factors obviously affect these findings. But there is clearly a correlation between high testosterone levels in women and an increased desire for independence at midlife, not to mention the high divorce rate among couples in their forties.

All the more reason, then, for recasting sex roles and experimenting a little. In time, polarization will occur if there is no give and take in the relationship, or if the newly revised sexual needs of both partners are not being met.

Laurie comments:

At first, I thought there was something wrong with my partner, that he was slowing down, losing his grip for some physical reason. This happened about the same time I seemed to want sex to be more physically forceful than before: faster, rougher, more intense. I found myself getting impatient with Ken, wishing he'd get on with it, at the same time feeling bad for being so pushy and demanding. But damn, what I wanted felt right to me, and I didn't want to put on the brakes.

This is a good start; the feeling is genuine and fits with the natural shift at this time. But there will be a breakdown without frank communication, understanding, and mutual support. If you are partnered with a man, and he wants time to warm up, choose your favorite foreplay and spell it out, loud and clear. If he is pacing himself to the utmost, initiate changes in position that keep the stimulation level high enough for you. Bring your fantasies into the picture. And don't be surprised if he is the one wanting afterglow cuddling and pillow talk!

The positive side of this shift is illustrated by these words from Candace:

> We'd been together for twelve years, and I finally felt like our sex life was fully on track. We truly understood where the other was coming from, because we'd each pretty much been there ourselves— we'd run the gamut, I guess. Sex just got better and better, and we had an erotic dimension in our communication that I remembered from the early stages of our relationship. It surprised me, exceeded my expectations, and was well worth waiting for.

This may also be a time when women seek intimate relationships with other women for the first time, based on common needs and desires. As Lynn reports:

> I never considered myself bisexual, never thought of being with a woman until I reached a place of certainty and confidence in myself that made me long for the affinity of an equal. I'd been with so many men, struggling with their problems. Then I fell in love with Susan, and found common life experience, humor, flexibility, and passion perfect for this time of my life.

In the next chapter, we will look at the transformative effects of menopause on a woman's life and sexuality.

CHAPTER 7

Sexual Transformation
in Menopause

Attitudes toward menopause in our society are mixed at best. Menopause not only signals the end of fertility but also is notorious for its physical and emotional side effects. Hot flashes hit unexpectedly, vaginal dryness can be distressing, and mood swings make us scream and cry as if we were in our teens. If our difficulties in accepting "the change" lead us to fight against it, these side effects often become increasingly extreme.

Compounding menopausal symptoms is our cultural bias against aging, particularly toward women, who often find themselves bereft of identity as they grow older. No wonder we approach menopause with a sense of dread! But there are ways to view this passage that afford us greater dignity and self-respect so that its benefits, not the least of which are sexual, may be celebrated and enjoyed.

At age forty-eight, I was the first of my women's circle to enter menopause. This was difficult, because even though my friends were close behind, I was moving into uncharted territory and felt isolated. Our discussions on the topic focused mostly on my symptoms, with ideas for herbs, dietary changes, or comfort measures that might help. Occasionally I talked about shifts in my sexuality, but with little clarity. I knew I was changing, but I didn't know how, and I certainly didn't know where I was going. After some months, I was finally able to express my frustration: "I don't want to know about this remedy or that, I want to know what is *happening* to me!"

Before long, I became so alarmed by my volatile moods and changing priorities that I decided to call for a Menopause Council in my community. There were five women I met with socially but didn't know well; they called themselves alternately "The Hot Potatoes," "The Fried Potatoes," or, "The Wild Yams." I asked one who was adept at women's circling if she would be willing to organize the council, and she agreed.

Soon I received an announcement for an event titled "The Other Side of Menopause." Each of the five organizers included a brief bio, and I was repeatedly struck by their third-person descriptions of how menopause had changed their lives:

> *She stopped bleeding at fifty-two, flipped the dial, and started listening to Her Own Voice.*

> *She last bled when she was fifty-three and has been expressing Grandmother's Voice of Wisdom and Truth.*

> *She stopped bleeding at forty-two after her uterus was removed and has since plunged into the well of grief, amazed to find laughter there as well as tears.*

> *She stopped bleeding when she was fifty, walked through a menopause door and met herself, and has become "Queen of her Own Country."*

> *She last bled when she was fifty-one, is her own Wild Darling, and the Heroine of Her Own Story.*

The effect of that council was far reaching for me and the forty other women who participated. Many of my fears were laid to rest, as I began to understand the scope of menopause as a major life passage. I learned that my experience of feeling out of sync with normal responsibilities was common, and I was reassured that the physical and emotional turmoil I felt was healthy. I also began to see that the sexual revolution going on inside me actually had a purpose.

What Is Menopause?

◎

At puberty, a girl has approximately three hundred thousand egg-forming cells, but a woman who is approaching menopause has only eight thousand or so follicles remaining. Over time, her eggs have been destroyed by a combination of stress, radiation (exposure to the sun), and normal degeneration. As eggs decrease in number, ovulation may not occur. And unless an egg ripens, there will be no corpus luteum to release progesterone (the first hormone to diminish). Even though the pituitary puts out increased amounts of FSH and LH, the ovaries become less responsive and their production of estrogen eventually ceases, as does menstruation.

Menopause occurs on average between the ages of forty-eight and fifty-two, although some women stop menstruating in their late thirties. Regardless of age, women typically experience four to six years when hormone levels progressively decline before menstruation ends, known as perimenopause. Many of the symptoms of this phase are caused by sharp fluctuations in levels of progesterone. Estrogen levels diminish slowly, but if no egg ripens in a given cycle, progesterone drops abruptly. This causes fluctuations in cycle length, intermittent bleeding, and greater blood loss with menstruation. Typically, periods are closer together and much heavier than before: Bleeding for a week to ten days is not unusual.

Problems can develop if cumulative blood loss becomes excessive. Sometimes a D&C is recommended to rule out uterine cancer. Fibroids and polyps may be implicated, but in the vast majority of cases, the problem is simply that progesterone levels are not high enough to maintain the uterine lining. Changes in diet and lifestyle, along with herbal remedies, may provide some relief. Studies show that deficiencies of iron, vitamin C, and bioflavonoids can exacerbate heavy bleeding, as can smoking, stress, and excessive intake of alcohol.

Some women experience less volatile decreases in progesterone and simply notice that their periods come less often and are lighter than before. They maybe troubled by symptoms of decreased estrogen, though—hot flashes, mood swings, night sweats, and vaginal changes. Again, nutritional and/or herbal remedies may help (see specific sections on each of these symptoms later in the chapter).

When a woman has stopped menstruating for a full year, her menopause is complete. This is the classic time for a menopause celebration (or Croning Rite; see the boxed section on page 175).

The age at which menopause occurs is somewhat hereditary; if your mother or sisters were later or earlier than usual, you are likely to follow suit. The average is now age fifty-one; at the turn of the century it was forty-six. Considering that life expectancy then was little more than fifty years, it is easy to see the basis of the fear that menopause marks the beginning of the end. But today, a woman can expect to live an average of eighty years, finishing menopause with more than a third of her life still ahead of her.

What will this last third of her life be like? Is she doomed, as the media would have us believe, to be shriveled and sexless, a doddery "senior citizen"? This largely depends on how well she takes care of herself physically, and on how she defines herself both personally and socially. But first, she must find a way to make it through "the change."

In the not so distant past, male authorities on the subject were harbingers of doom. Robert A. Wilson, author of *Feminine Forever* and staunch advocate of hormone replacement therapy (HRT), described menopause as "the loss of womanhood and the loss of good health," claiming that "chemical imbalances" result in "castration and a state of living decay."[1] David Reuben, author of *Everything You Always Wanted to Know About Sex but Were Afraid to Ask,* also saw menopause as the end for women: "Having outlived their ovaries, they may have outlived their usefulness as human beings. The remaining years may just be marking time until they follow their glands into oblivion."[2]

But women experts today have other opinions. Sheila Kitzinger views menopause as a process by which "a new balance is found, one which is natural and right for an older woman." She is quick to point out that although estrogen and progesterone diminish, increased testosterone more than compensates.[3] Susan Lark, author of *The Menopause Self-Help Book,* notes that because women tend to pay better attention to their health in menopause than ever before, these years can be a time of unprecedented "vigor and vitality."[4] Or, as author Susan Love humorously reminds us, "Your ovaries aren't quitting, they're changing careers, just like the rest of you."[5]

The key is to view menopause as a natural, but major, life transition. It is a period of intense and incontrovertible change, marked by emotional and physical extremes much as in the transition phase of labor, the postpartum period, or the premenstrual phase of the monthly cycle. In all of these, equilibrium is found not by struggling for control, but by surrendering to the change and seeing it through. Coping techniques for PMS, labor, or postpartum can help in menopause, but trust in the process largely determines the ease of its progression.

Much has been said already of how difficult it can be to let go this way. Our culture so expects female constancy that we may deny ourselves opportunities to experience the heights and depths of life as men do, whether by acts of creativity or foolishness, courage or delusion. Nevertheless, a dance of extremes takes place in our flesh, patterned hormonally in our monthly cycle and our Blood Mysteries. Particularly with the latter, we have little choice but to go wild.

Inherent in our wild times is a chance to take stock of ourselves, to assess where we have been and where we have yet to go. Comments like "I no longer love my career" or "I feel alone in my primary relationship" are typical in menopause and hold keys to new directions for the next part life. Sweeping changes can and should occur at this time. It is foolish not to use the menopause transition for a few radical departures and explorations into the unknown.

Dr. Christiane Northrup and Mona Lisa Schulz have written extensively on changes in brain function during menopause. In their research, they found levels of FSH and LH to be approximately a thousand times greater than at any other point in the lifecycle. At first glance, this information is confounding—why would the pituitary bother to produce so much FSH and LH at a time when these substances have no apparent function? It turns out that FSH and LH have a very different effect in menopausal woman than in women who are cycling—they serve as neurotransmitters in the right side of the brain, the hemisphere associated with creativity, intuition, and visionary experience.[6]

What a revelation! One of the main reasons I called for a Menopause Council was that I was having an increasing number of intuitive, visionary experiences in my daily life, which I believed must be somehow connected to menopause. That day, I shared that I had gone nine months with no period, but when I unexpectedly bled again it was as if a curtain fell in front of my eyes—the exquisite visionary dimension I had been exploring just slipped away. Northrup and Schulz's research makes clear that menopause truly is a time when women become wise, if only they can trust the process.

Thus any aspect of our past that we have difficulty releasing can make menopausal symptoms worse. In this way, dealing with menopause is similar to coping with PMS. Although some of our premenstrual outbursts are of little consequence, the *intensity* of these outbursts may reveal how much we are holding in or holding back. The same is true in menopause. In my research, I've found that menopausal women are almost compulsive in their need to get on with their lives, find new work, start new relationships, or do whatever is necessary to be intimate with their truth.

Physical Symptoms and Treatment

◎

Hormonal symptoms of menopause include hot flashes, heart palpitations, night sweats, and itching of the skin. Effects include vaginal dryness, bladder dysfunction, joint pain, muscle weakness, wrinkling of the skin, thinning of the hair, weight gain, bloating, headache, and osteoporosis. Emotional reactions include moodiness and irritability, insomnia, forgetfulness, and changes in sexual desire. Guidelines for coping with these symptoms fall more or less into one of two camps: obliteration of symptoms through hormonal control, or cooperation with the process via health-enhancing practices.

Keep in mind that hormone replacement therapy (HRT) was developed by physicians. Ignorant and fearful of women's bodies, they perceived menopause, as well as birth and menstruation, to be abnormal conditions in need of treatment or medication. To illustrate: One of my students recounted that her mother, in labor and at the height of transition, called her doctor a "goddamn son-of-a-bitch" and was sedated without her consent.

Certainly in our culture, men are unprepared to deal with women's biological transitions, particularly when at full throttle, and have thus sought ways to dominate and control women at these junctures. Medication is a powerful way to do this. This is not to discount the value of hormone replacement in certain circumstances, but the routine use of hormones to address common complaints of menopause is just as bad as drugging the body in childbirth or obliterating premenstrual symptoms with antidepressants.

As author Joan Borysenko wryly notes in *Reflections on a Woman's Book of Life*, our solution for women's "irrational" behavior is to put them on oral contraceptives at menarche, take them off long enough for childbearing, medicate them for birth, get them back on oral contraceptives until menopause, and then start HRT. How would it be, she wonders, if we had a medication for men, we'll call it "test-away," that could similarly be started at adolescence, stopped briefly for child siring, then continued on through old age? Think how calm and compliant men would be, she muses—no wild drinking, crazy driving, fights, and so on.

What made HRT attractive to women in the first place? When HRT was first developed, it was touted as the only way menopausal women might stay youthful. It was marketed as a panacea for sleeplessness, depression, loss of interest in sex, dry skin and hair, fatigue—in other words, all the undesired effects of aging.

But now the data is in, and the benefits of HRT are questionable at best. Even though estrogen may help reduce hot flashes, vaginal changes, and wrinkling of the skin, and progesterone may treat excessive bleeding, conjugated (synthetic) forms of these hormones have been shown to have serious side effects and contraindications. In one study, HRT increased the rate of breast cancer by 26 percent.[7] If synthetic estrogen is used exclusively (ERT) for six or more years, the risk of uterine cancer is increased ten times, as are risks for gall bladder disease, stroke, thrombosis, phlebitis, headaches, and depression: It is contraindicated for anyone suffering from liver disease, sickle cell anemia, gall stones, diabetes, or abnormal vaginal bleeding.[8]

What about the long-touted benefits of HRT in reducing heart disease? On the contrary, the Women's Health Initiative study showed a 22 percent *increase* in cardiovascular disease with HRT.[9]

Northrup maintains that increased insulin resistance, present in 50 to 75 percent of women, is the number one factor in the development of heart disease. A 1977 study published in the *American Journal of Clinical Nutrition* showed that a high-carbohydrate, excessively low-fat diet put women at risk, deleteriously affecting lipid and insulin levels in the body.[10]

Although physicians are increasingly aware of this information, any woman on HRT must make her own decision. If she has had surgical removal of the ovaries or hysterectomy, particularly if under the age of forty, HRT may ease the transition to an early menopause. Still, she must be alert to signs of estrogen overdose, as each of us has our own level of tolerance: These include water retention, folic acid anemia, bloating, nausea, and breast tenderness. Signs of progesterone excess include increased susceptibility to vaginal yeast and other infections, fatigue, and hirsutism (excess body and facial hair).

As depression is a known side effect of HRT, an antidepressant may be added to the formula. But depression with HRT is most often due to insufficient testosterone, which leads to lowered libido and a flat emotional affect (much as is true of women on the Pill). Psychologist Barbara Sherwin of McGill of the University in Montreal demonstrated this in her research on women who experienced early menopause due to hysterectomy. Compared to those taking estrogen and progesterone only, women whose formulas included testosterone had more intense sexual desires and fantasies, were more easily aroused, and had orgasms more frequently. They also had higher energy levels and a greater sense of well-being.[11]

Antidepressant use for women not on HRT seems misguided, at best, as most studies show menopausal women to be no more inherently depressed than women at other stages of life. But again, the explosive emotions of this period often lead to a prescription. Rosetta Reitz, author of *Menopause: A Positive Approach,* believes this to be a strategy to keep women at this stage out of sight and out of mind. "Do you know what would happen if all the women between forty and fifty-five started making demands?" she queries. "My adrenaline begins to burst forth at the excitement of the idea." Other drawbacks to antidepressants include chemical dependency and the interruption of REM sleep, which is necessary for dreaming.

Although testosterone dips naturally in menopause, it soon

returns to previous levels and continues to rise steadily as we age. Herbs such as nettle stimulate the adrenals to produce adequate testosterone. Red raspberry leaf and hawthorn berry teas invigorate the system and help alleviate depression, as can St. John's wort. But stress reduction, or doing whatever is necessary to eliminate chronic stress, is the key. As Rollin McCraty (director of research for the Institute for HeartMath) reminds us, finding appreciation in life and thinking with the heart changes its beat-to-beat variability in such a way that more DHEA is produced, which is the precursor to testosterone.[12]

Decreased levels of testosterone in menopause can be distressing, but may serve to refocus us on larger issues in our lives. This account serves to illustrate:

> *I've pretty well completed my menopause, I'm beginning to get my energy back, and I'm not feeling the childlike things I felt earlier in my passage. The emotional swings were very much like adolescence—I would feel things explosively, and tears came very easily. For me, this was all part of seeing my attachment to my body, and learning just what my body is and isn't. For instance, my libido went way down, and I've always had a very strong sex drive—it was just like falling off a cliff. I had sworn that I would be vibrantly sexual till my dying day, and when I discovered how much of that urge was really physiological and driven by hormones, I felt a little bit of... almost embarrassment at my presumption, thinking I knew myself and realizing that what I had identified as self was so much physical. At that point, a lot of things just started falling away, my attachment to relationship and the feeling of protection I'd had by having another person around. I began to see my strength as coming from my own centeredness, centeredness in Spirit.[13]*

As we look more closely at specific menopausal symptoms and their potential effect on sexuality, we will consider the use of herbs, supplements, and dietary changes to address these concerns. (For more-detailed information, see the chart on the next page.)

Symptoms in Menopause and Their Treatment

Symptom(s)	Nutritional Supplements	Natural Sources
Excess bleeding	Vitamin A 5,000 IU	Hawthorn berry, vitex
	Vitamin C 1,000 mg	Dandelion root
	Iron 30 mg	Shepherd's purse
	Bioflavonoids 800 mg	Black haw, false unicorn, sarsaparilla, wild yam root
Hot flashes	Vitamin E 800 IU	Motherwort
	Bioflavonoids 800 mg	Black cohosh, dong quai, fennel, pomegranate
Vaginal changes	Vitamin E 800 IU	Motherwort
	Bioflavonoids 800 mg	Saw palmetto berries
	Evening primrose oil	Comfrey ointment
	Linseed oil	
Urinary tract problems	Vitamin C 1,000–1,500 mg	Black currant, goldenseal, nettle, uva ursi, yarrow
Osteoporosis	Vitamin D 5,000 IU	Oat straw
	Calcium citrate 1,500 mg	Nettle
	Folic acid 800 mcg	Comfrey root
	Zinc 20 mg	Horsetail
	Magnesium 500 mg	
Nervous irritability	Vitamin B complex 50 mg	Passionflower
	Vitamin C 1,000 mg	Valerian root
	Bioflavonoids 800 mg	Catnip, hops
Fatigue, depression	Vitamin B complex 50 mg	Ginger
	Vitamin C 1,000 mg	Cayenne pepper
	Magnesium 500 mg	Oat straw
	Potassium aspartate 100 mg	Blessed thistle

Hot Flashes

Three out of four women experience hot flashes, the most common menopausal symptom. Hot flashes are the only symptom considered to be universal, occurring among women in virtually every culture. During a hot flash, there is a rush of heat to the chest, neck, and face, or sometimes the entire body. This can happen anytime, anywhere. The skin reddens, temperature increases, and breathing becomes shallow. There may also be an itching sensation. As the heat passes, women often find themselves drenched in sweat, and may then feel chilly and drained. These episodes may or may not be noticed by others; regardless, women are often disoriented or embarrassed by them.

Hot flashes are linked to decreasing estrogen, and also to high levels of LH. The precise mechanism of their occurrence remains unknown. Some women never experience hot flashes; others have them three times a day or more. Many experience them only at night. The hot flashes and night sweats of menopause are very much like those experienced postpartum, due also to hormonal fluctuations. Hot flashes usually persist no more than five years: Most women have them for several months only.

Physically, hot flashes result from vasomotor instability originating in the temperature-regulating center of the hypothalamus. Some women are so susceptible that even subtle temperature changes caused by exercise, stress, sexual arousal, or cold or hot room environments can trigger them. Others note a strong correlation between hot flashes and drinking caffeinated beverages or alcohol. Large doses of niacin (vitamin B-6) and certain drugs, such as those used to treat hypertension, are also implicated. Emotional upsets can trigger hot flashes, too.

Commonsense measures include layering clothing so that certain items can be shed quickly, keeping a spray bottle by the bed, in the car, and at the office, having a change of sheets or towels by the bed, and using a small electric fan when feasible. Although supplemental estrogen can control hot flashes, they come right back when treatment is stopped. Tincture of motherwort, twenty drops under the tongue, is reputed to be one of the best natural remedies. Tincture of black cohosh works well, too. Soy products (organic, not GMO) are extremely effective; soy is an excellent source of plant-based phytoestrogens, which are readily absorbed without negative side effects. Bioflavonoids added to the diet or taken as a supplement can help, too. Homeopathic remedies may also be useful, lachesis in particular. For more information on this and other therapies, see *New Menopausal Years: The Wise Woman Way*, by Susun Weed. This is a comprehensive and inspiring book; one of my favorites.[14]

Apart from the nuisance, some women view hot flashes as an opportunity to change their perspective. Many of my clients speak of surrendering to their flashes and feeling stimulated or illuminated. Some say that hot flashes trigger intuitive insights and revelations. Barbara Raskin, author of *Hot Flashes*, describes these messages as "urgent communiqués from the interior of a vast, dark continent... fast-breaking news items from my heart of darkness."[15] Darkness is the medium of the Crone, who weaves the web of life and cuts away that which has outlived its usefulness. Hot flashes provide a metaphysical opportunity to connect with the shadow side of our nature and use it to let go of whatever we don't need in our lives anymore.

Women also find that the better they get to know themselves in menopause, the more likely they are to know when a hot flash is coming. Sometimes a revelation precedes the flash and may thus serve as a signal to take off a sweater or turn on the fan. At the most basic level, hot flashes result from overload of the endocrine system, which is busy adjusting multiple physiological functions to match changed levels of estrogen and progesterone. Overload equals altered state, and that is exactly what hot flashes initiate.

Kitzinger likens the process of coping with hot flashes to that of coping with labor contractions. She recommends slowing down and opening up, breathing from low in the body, down in the pelvis.

This can change the experience from upsetting to erotic. We can use our hot flashes to heighten awareness in a variety of ways, depending on how we focus our attention.

Vaginal and Pelvic Changes

In menopause, vaginal tissues may thin and become easily damaged. There may be a lack of lubrication as well, caused by a reduction of transvaginal electropotential (the mechanism by which water and electrolytes are conveyed across vaginal tissues). For most women, this is temporary and does not affect libido, but it can certainly influence sex itself.

These changes occur as estrogen levels drop prior to the creation of a new hormonal balance. The vagina becomes more alkaline than usual and hence more vulnerable to infection. Decreased estrogen can also lead to reduced vaginal and pelvic circulation, implicating the bladder and accounting for the increased incidence of urinary tract infections.

Of all the symptoms of menopause for which estrogen therapy is suggested, vaginal dryness is the one for which it is most widely used. But suppositories of vitamin E are a fine alternative. Lubricating jelly will still be necessary on occasion—try a lightweight, more natural feeling product, such as Astroglide. Note that seminal fluid has a positive effect on vaginal tissues as does evening primrose oil: Both contain prostaglandins, which soften and condition. Orgasm is also beneficial; according to Rosetta Reitz, intercourse and masturbation on a regular basis make vaginal and pelvic changes at menopause "hardly noticeable." One study showed that weekly intercourse so increased women's estrogen levels that these changes and other common complaints due to estrogen deficiency were eliminated.[16]

As already discussed, continued use of estrogen alone carries significant health risks; therefore, natural alternatives should be utilized. Besides the lubricants mentioned above, the addition of soy products (as defined above) can help. Vitamin E, at least 600 IU taken daily, helps too. Bioflavonoids are important as well: Take approximately 800 mg daily, or eat more citrus fruit (especially the inner rind) and buckwheat. Herbal teas of licorice root and black cohosh root also help stimulate estrogen production.

For urinary tract problems, herbs like goldenseal and uva ursi (bearberry) are classic. Goldenseal contains berberine, which has antibiotic affects, and uva ursi has arbutin, a diuretic and anti-infective agent. The two can be combined and simmered slowly to make a tea, or may be taken as tincture. And the classic recommendation of pure cranberry juice or capsules works because a substance it contains, proanthocyanadin, prevents bacteria from adhering to uroepithelial cells. See the boxed text on pages 166–168 for additional ideas.

Osteoporosis

The term *osteoporosis* refers to a loss of bone mass, and although it occurs in men, it is more common among women in our culture. Estrogen plays a critical role in maintaining the structure and calcification of bone, so the decline in this hormone at menopause is thought to precipitate the condition. But there are other factors involved. Genetic predisposition figures strongly in osteoporosis, as does a diet high in salt, animal protein, caffeine, alcohol, or carbonated drinks (high levels of phosphorus directly decrease bone mass). Some authorities feel that inadequate intake of vitamin D may be a primary factor, particularly as exposure to sunlight is increasingly discouraged. This is corroborated by cross-cultural studies showing that osteoporosis is far from universal in menopausal women. Some populations show no osteoporosis in women at any age, while in others both men and women are affected, even prior to midlife. The incidence is definitely higher in industrialized countries, among women who smoke, have a Northern European background, are sedentary, or regularly use drugs such as steroids, diuretics, aluminum-containing antacids, thyroid supplements, and anticonvulsants.

The effects of osteoporosis are worse than the condition itself. The spine tends to compress and curve, and certain bones, particularly the hips, are highly susceptible to fracture. Such injuries usually occur later in life, around ages seventy to eighty. Thirty percent of women thus affected die of complications, and many more suffer chronic disability.

It seems obvious that diet and lifestyle are major factors in osteoporosis. What are some of the ways we can prevent this condition? First, we must stop worrying about the extra five or ten pounds typically gained at menopause, and start focusing more on nutrition (ideally, long before menopause occurs). There is evidence that our ability to absorb calcium from dairy products decreases with age, so we must find other sources. Calcium citrate, found almost exclusively in products like orange juice with added calcium, is much more readily absorbed than is calcium lactate. Dark leafy green vegetables and seeds, especially sesame, are fine sources too.

Calcium is, however, just one of many nutrients essential to good health. An optimal diet for menopause should consist of plenty of green and yellow vegetables, legumes, fresh fruit in season, complex carbohydrates, nuts and seeds, and moderate amounts of grass-fed beef, cage-free chicken, and fish from unpolluted waters (an excellent source of the omega fatty acids). Particularly important are trace minerals, but these are often leached from the soil by commercial farming methods. Organic fruits and vegetables are as much as five times higher in nutritional value than their commercial counterparts. It is definitely worth finding a store that stocks organic produce.[17] See the boxed text starting on the next page for more details on nutrition in menopause.

Supplements can also help increase or maintain bone density. Calcium, magnesium, boron, vitamin C, and vitamin D all play crucial roles in preventing osteoporosis. If diagnosed with osteoporosis, natural progesterone cream works well for many women.

~~~ Nutrition in Menopause* ~~~

Good nutrition is of utmost importance during menopause. As we age, the digestive tract produces fewer enzymes and less hydrochloric acid, a condition further exacerbated by stress. Yet many menopausal problems and complaints can be minimized or alleviated by eating the right foods.

Whole Grains

Whole grains include whole organic corn and wheat, quinoa, unhulled barley, oats, rye, millet, buckwheat, brown rice, and wild rice. They stabilize blood sugar levels and reduce sugar cravings. They also help to prevent diabetes and may also protect against cancer of the colon, as they are high in fiber. Eat freely of these, and try for some variety each week. Raw wheat germ is a good source of vitamin E, helpful for vaginal dryness and other low estrogen symptoms.

Legumes

Legumes are the peas and beans, such as lentils, kidney beans, black beans, chickpeas, pinto beans, white beans, and split peas. All are high in protein and fiber and digest slowly, making them especially appropriate for older women. Problems with gas can be alleviated by slow and thorough cooking, or by eating smaller amounts.

Vegetables

Vegetables provide a full range of vitamins and minerals. The dark green, orange, and red varieties are high in vitamin A, which has been shown to protect against cancer of the breast and cervix, as well as immunological disease. Vitamin C has similar benefits and also helps prevent excessive bleeding at menopause if combined with iron and bioflavonoids. Good

Partially adapted from *The Menopause Self-Help Book* by Susan Lark, MD   (cont'd.)
(Berkeley, CA: Celestial Arts, 2004).

sources of vitamin C include peppers, potatoes, peas, tomatoes, broccoli, cabbage, parsley, and kale. Vegetables also provide important minerals such as calcium, magnesium, iron, zinc, copper, and trace elements, especially if grown organically. Onions and garlic help lower serum cholesterol, reducing the risk of strokes and heart attacks. Seaweeds such as kelp and nori are high in iodine, which promotes healthy thyroid function.

Fruits

Fruits also provide a wide range of vitamins and minerals. They are especially rich in potassium, which serves to regulate blood pressure. Potassium also helps prevent the fatigue commonly associated with menopause: Good sources are bananas, berries, melons, grapefruit, peaches, and apricots. High fiber content is yet another bonus of eating fresh fruit, alleviating constipation. Pineapple and papaya specifically aid digestion by breaking down proteins.

Seeds and Nuts

Seeds and nuts are good sources of protein, but they are very high in fat and calories and thus should be eaten sparingly. Magnesium, potassium, and calcium are quite concentrated in nuts and seeds, particularly almonds, sunflower seeds, pumpkin seeds, and sesame seeds. They digest best if eaten raw, ground into meal or butter.

Fish and Poultry

Red meats laden with hormones and preservatives must be avoided. Fish from unpolluted waters and organic poultry are preferred sources of animal protein. Fish is an outstanding source of linoleic acid, which can help with dryness of the hair, skin, and vaginal tissues (this may also be taken

(cont'd.)

supplementally as linseed oil, in liquid or capsule form). Fish is also a good source of the omega fatty acids, known to help prevent neurological problems associated with age, such as Alzheimer's disease.

Foods to Avoid

Note that this section repeatedly refers to excess amount of these items; moderation is the key.

Salt

In excess, salt can exacerbate bloating, high blood pressure, heart disease, and osteoporosis.

Sugar

Too much refined sweetener can accelerate diabetes, deplete essential vitamins and minerals, and cause stress, anxiety, and vulnerability to infection.

Caffeine

Excess caffeine can cause mood swings, interfere with carbohydrate metabolism, exacerbate hot flashes, and worsen osteoporosis.

Alcohol

Alcohol has similar effects to those of caffeine. It also disrupts the liver's ability to metabolize hormones, intensifying menopausal complaints.

Fats

Polyunsaturated and hydrogenated vegetable oils, found in processed foods and high in trans-fats, must be avoided as they are correlated to heart disease, high blood pressure, stroke, and cancer of the ovaries, breasts, and uterus. Substitute healthy fats found in organic meat, fish, and poultry; avocado; and nuts and seeds.

(cont'd.)

An over busy or sedentary lifestyle also has negative effects. Most of us spend way too much time indoors, sitting at a desk or doing housework that keeps us just this side of aerobic, chronically tense with the pressure of having so many things to do. This is the opposite of what we need: good food, regular exercise, and daily relaxation in complementary measure. In fact, next to getting enough calcium in the diet, the single most important way to avoid osteoporosis is with weight-bearing exercise: basically, any upright activity such as walking, dancing, bicycling, climbing stairs, or lifting free weights. As women, we are especially apt to defer to the needs of others and may thus deprive ourselves of these health-promoting necessities. Eventually, and sometimes with surprising swiftness, this can catch up with us.

It's a good idea to ask your mother or older sisters what menopause was like for them, because patterns and severity of symptoms tend to be somewhat hereditary. Even more important are the coping mechanisms your female relatives used: What worked and what didn't. I was relieved when my mother told me menopause had been a breeze for her; she had occasional hot flashes and that was about it. But if your family history is not so rosy, don't panic. Get the full picture, making sure to factor in the effects of pharmaceutical interventions and lifestyle before jumping to any conclusions.

Thus far, we've considered menopause primarily as a natural phenomenon. When it is surgically induced, as by hysterectomy, the experience is very different. Instead of a gradual decline in hormonal levels, a woman experiences abrupt withdrawal—her system is thrown into shock.

By age sixty, approximately one in three women in the United States will have had a hysterectomy, the highest rate for any country in the world. Fifty-five percent are performed on women ages thirty-five to forty-nine.[18] Many gynecologists still believe that women beyond their childbearing prime are safer without their reproductive organs: "the uterus is for growing babies or for growing cancer."[19] This viewpoint utterly discounts the physical difficulties and emotional trauma women typically experience when meno-pause occurs so abruptly. Even when there are clear indications for surgery, a woman's loss of her reproductive organs can cause deep depression and grief (see Chapter 9).

There are four main indications for hysterectomy: (1) cancer of the reproductive organs; (2) severe infection of the fallopian tubes, uterus, or ovaries that cannot be controlled; (3) extremely large fi-broid tumors; and (4) uncontrollable uterine bleeding unrespon-sive to D&C or any other remedy. Yet these conditions account for only 12 percent of all hysterectomies, indicating that most hysterec-tomies are unnecessary.

If hysterectomy is recommended for fibroids or uterine bleed-ing, the ovaries do not have to be removed, particularly if the woman is over forty, when her risk of ovarian cancer drops to one percent. Subtotal hysterectomy, whereby the ovaries or some part thereof are saved, is always best because even a small portion of a single ovary can continue hormonal production. If the difficulty is fibroids alone, a myomectomy may permit surgical removal of the fibroid while saving the uterus. Although fibroid tissue tends to grow back, myomectomy is the best solution for the woman whose fibroid has grown cumbersome and who still desires children.

As mentioned earlier, symptoms of surgically induced meno-pause are usually so extreme as to necessitate HRT, at least for a while. Many women try to taper their formula down to a minimal level by their late forties and discontinue in the fifties: a wise deci-sion, considering the well-documented side effects of HRT.

Sex for the woman who has undergone complete hysterectomy is apt to be distressing both physically and emotionally. Annette re-calls:

I felt empty, like I had nothing to offer anymore. My muscles were all shot and soft—my vagina was foreign territory to me and I wasn't sure I wanted to get to know it again. Having to face the fact that I'd never have a child and would never give birth was unspeakably painful to me, and stole the magic from sex and my body for a very long time.

Another woman reports:

The inside of me felt all stopped up and rigid—like a dead end, literally. I had periodic bleeding at first, which was normal, they said. Even though it was scary, I actually welcomed it—at least something was coming out of me! When I bled, I found that I could cry. After it stopped, I turned my sadness inward until I healed.

On the other side, here's an account from Mandy:

I had suffered so much with endometriosis and recurrent uterine infection that the decision for hysterectomy came as a relief. I wasn't sure I wanted kids anyway, and now the matter was settled. But I noticed a funny thing: For months after the surgery, I still felt a rhythm, a ghost cycle I guess. I didn't know how much that rhythm had become a part of me, wracked with pain as I was.

Some women notice a change in orgasms after hysterectomy. The deep contractions felt in the uterus, or the stimulation of the cervix that some women find so pleasurable, are no longer part of the experience. This sort of sexual crisis necessitates refocusing and reconditioning oneself (and one's partner) to find satisfaction in other pleasure centers.

Brooke Medicine Eagle, a Native-American authority on women's health issues, speaks frequently on the meaning of surgical menopause. She speculates that hysterectomy in the childbearing years may afford certain women the opportunity to assume mature leadership roles traditionally held by their elders, due to our deficit in women's wisdom and the urgent need for its resurgence. In her tradition, whenever and however menopause occurs, it marks a time when a woman retains her precious menstrual fluid or "wise blood" for increased awareness and greater wisdom. Postmenopausal women of the "Grandmother Lodge" are thus accorded the deepest respect and the highest honor.[20]

Sex During Menopause

◎

What is sex like at this time? Reports range wildly, from plain disinterest to blooming desire. Decreased testosterone levels, although temporary, may put a damper on passion, but so can emotional revelations. From Marjorie:

> *Looking back, I think my moodiness had a lot to do with it. I never really let go of wanting to have a second child, even though the years went by and nothing happened. Then menopause put an end to that dream, and I cried and raged at my husband, to the point that he called the doctor for sedatives! I tried estrogen for a while but just got more depressed. I wanted absolutely nothing to do with Blake...I acted as though it was all his fault. And I really did blame him—when I wanted kids early in our marriage, he wasn't ready, and then we had to wait so long for our son. Anyway, my hot flashes were awful, they happened to me everywhere and often made me cry. Sometimes I'd come home and scream in the closet, when no one was around.*
>
> *We didn't have sex, except once in a while when I felt I could stomach it, like once a month or so. After it [menopause] was all over, though, I got my drive back all right...I only wish my husband had. Things are different between us now...I guess we'll never be the same.*

Quite the opposite experience, from Geri:

> *Menopause was liberation for me. I didn't expect it, but so it was. No more worries about birth control—after four children, free at last! By then, the youngest was almost grown. I took classes at the local college, art and creative writing. I felt so good to finally be able to go after my dreams. And sex, well, we reached new heights with it. My drive became more intense, my confidence increased, my husband loved it! He began to take more time with me, feeding my senses and enjoying my rhythms. We were really on a par.*

Geri's story is actually a bit more postmenopausal. Here is Elaine's tale, from deep in the thick of it:

I welcomed menopause; I wasn't afraid because I'd learned to trust my body over the years and felt ready for whatever it had in store for me. The intensity of the hot flashes threw me at first, but I began to see them as a sort of release. When I looked at menopause as a transition to my wiser, seasoned self, I decided that with every flash, I'd let something go, some obligation to someone else's priorities, some outdated idea of myself, some old wound. It was exhilarating to do this—really a rush! Sometimes I'd flash during lovemaking, usually at the beginning of arousal, and I'd use it to boost my passion. My partner had no complaints. He didn't always know what was up, but sex often took the edge off my sharpness. Menopausal women are so powerful—I think men can be intimated by the change. For us, sex was the bridge.

Diane says this of her experience with Elsa:

I was in menopause before my partner, by about a year or so. We both experienced hot flashes for a while, although hers were usually more intense. It was fun, and really wonderful for both of us to have the support and understanding. Minor inconveniences some women speak of, like vaginal dryness—applying oils to each other just became part of our sexual pleasure. But the dimension menopause opened for us was the big surprise…we had always been telepathic to some extent, but now we could read each other with ease.

Last, a classically mixed response:

I grieved during menopause—I hate to admit it, because I consider myself a modern woman—but I was deeply afraid of growing old, of losing my looks. This affected my self-confidence and desire for sex. I was afraid I'd lose my husband, so I shut down in bed—I was scared of being vulnerable. When my hot flashes were the most intense we stopped making love for a while, I guess for about three months or so. My vagina felt different too, drier and very tender. In retrospect, I think I was testing my husband, and lo and behold, after it was all over, he was still there. Then my desire skyrocketed, and I took hold of the situation.

Celebrating "the Change"

In Native-American and many other indigenous cultures, women at menopause are honored by rites that help them celebrate the event and more deeply appreciate its meaning. But menopause in our culture is often accompanied by feelings of sadness and uncertainty. What sort of ritual might we employ to help us acknowledge these feelings, while at the same time exploring the potential of this transition?

Most menopause rituals naturally incorporate practices for letting go of the past and welcoming new responsibilities. For example, women may gather around a fire (or a symbolic candle) and take turns, one by one, giving up some fear, resentment, or self-limiting belief to be consumed by the flame. If the fire is large enough, each woman can throw in a token of her surrender—a piece of wood, paper, cloth, or other symbolic item.

As each woman takes her turn, she speaks of her deepest lesson in life, and of that which she still intends to accomplish. Members of the group can acknowledge what she has said, and charge her with the responsibility of serving as the caretaker of life via her special gifts and vision. It's best to have women of all ages present at a menopause rite: the Crones (women in their wisdom years), Matriarchs (women in their power years), Mothers (women in their nurturing years), and Maidens (women in their innocent years).

In essence, the transition to Cronehood signifies a time when women transmute their personal pursuits and the demands of childbearing to become "keepers of the law." Their role shifts from nurturing their immediate families to caring for humanity. Their seasoned sense of justice and peacekeeping abilities are now available to society. The word *Crone* is actually similar in derivation to *crown,* signifying leadership. Even the word *hag,* which has such a derogatory meaning in our culture, comes from the Greek *hagia,* meaning "a holy one."[21]

In yet another ritual, everyone gathers around a large bowl or pot of water. Each has a cup, and moving clockwise, each takes a turn to dip and drink, saying, "I accept the wisdom of ages past." The Crones then form an inner circle. One begins by saying what she has learned in life, what wisdom she still seeks or what she must do to complete her life's mission. As she finishes, the Crone to her right reminds her, "Take from the wisdom of the ages the means to fulfill your destiny," or "Shed the skin that has become too tight for you and be born anew."[22]

When the Crones are done, the outer circle of women repeats the process. As each finishes speaking, the Crones respond in turn by repeating the one of the blessings given above.

Although these rituals work best in groups, the same acts of letting go of the past, naming life lessons, and identifying the keys to one's future may be done in solitude. Use a candle, water, or both, and be sure to give voice to your thoughts: The power of the spoken word is great. Also see the boxed section below.

The Croning Rite*

This rite of passage is observed when a woman has completed menopause, with no menstruation for a full year. The postmenopausal stage heralds the start of a new life phase, when she is to be venerated for her life experience. It is a time of celebration. Or, if a woman has undergone premature menopause due to surgical or chemical intervention, she may have her Croning ritual whenever she wants.

---

* Reprinted from *The Women's Wheel of Life* (revised) by Elizabeth Davis and Carol Leonard

(cont'd.)

Menopause honoring still occurs in non-industrial societies, but these rites are increasingly contaminated by patriarchal feelings of shame and disgust. This is why it is so
important to recreate these rites, lest they be obliterated.

In the Seneca tradition, a woman entering perimenopause speaks with the Grandmothers of her tribe and
chooses a subject to teach the young women of her community. Possible subjects include the spirituality of dreams,
animals, trees, or food. Or she may choose to address the
challenges of maturation for women and children. After
teaching for a year, she becomes a Grandmother and is revered as a wise one. When her menopause is finally complete, she is accorded the further honor of being allowed to
select the chiefs of her tribe.

Older women of some Jewish communities mark the
transition from mother to elder by changing their names. In
similar fashion, Native-American women at menopause are
often given new names by their chief.

The menopause rite is designed around a standard format. The woman's female friends and relations gather to deco-
rate the room, using evergreens, which signify immortality,
or other boughs of winter classically representing the Crone.
The ceremony can begin by weaving a "Mother Line:" as
participants pass a candle or ceremonial object around the
circle, each speaks her name and that of her mother, grandmother and great-grandmother, going back in her female
lineage as far as she can. "I am Susan, daughter of Caroline,
granddaughter of Rose, great-granddaughter of Violet."

The body of the rite can take various forms. I recall the
rite we held for a Crone midwife who was retiring from active practice. Each midwife in attendance shared a memory
of working with her, and as they told their stories they wove

(cont'd.)

red, white, and black yarn, along with some special trinket, into a "story belt." Some of the stories were hilarious, but the result was a poignant, ceremonial object of inestimable value. Or the women in the circle can take turns telling the Crone what it has meant to have her as a friend, or ask her an important personal question in hopes that, with her newfound authority, she will provide wise counsel. To close, a pomegranate is given to her and she is to ingest as many seeds as years she has lived, with as many blessings for continued fruitfulness in the years to come.

The Crone can conclude her rite privately, making time for personal contemplation. This aspect of seclusion is found in numerous other rites, and is symbolic of rebirth. It is best to do this part of the ritual at the dark moon or earliest crescent, as this lunar phase represents regeneration, a time of new beginnings. The Crone may make an offering to signify letting go of regrets and trusting what is yet to come. Meanwhile, her friends feast and make merry, and prepare to welcome her return with love, laughter, and feasting.

CHAPTER 8

Sex *in* Later Years

Just how satisfying a woman's sex life is once she is past menopause depends largely on how she retains her self-respect and zest for life. Against all odds, she must define her continued growth as valuable, despite society's views to the contrary. The image of older women as washed up or outmoded is so pervasive that this can be difficult indeed. Culturally, we value women mostly for their physical beauty and service to others. No wonder many women suffer as they age, as their children leave home, and as their family obligations lessen.

One of our finest references for tracking demeaning attitudes toward older women is Barbara Walker's *The Crone*. Walker documents that in pre-Christian societies worldwide, the mythic triumvirate of Virgin, Mother, and Crone reigned supreme. Christian mythology eliminated the Crone, retaining only the more benign and readily controlled Maiden and Mother figures.[1]

What made the Crone so threatening? In the Hindu tradition, she was known as Kali the Destroyer—not that she was maliciously violent or spiteful, but she did possess fierce instincts to terminate anything that had exhausted its usefulness so that it might be transformed to something new. Accordingly, her power was tremendous. In myth after myth, the Crone persona proved stronger than any god. As the Teutonic Elli, she conquered Thor, the god of strength.

As the Celtic Morgana Le Fay (or Morgan of the Fates), she had the power to humble and tame all men. As the Greek Atropos the Cutter, she snipped the thread of every life.

The aspect of the Crone most frightening to men of any age is her power to refuse to care for their personal concerns to the exclusion of her care for society at large. Women's power to say no, to see and serve a higher moral code or natural law, is what men have sought so persistently and desperately to obliterate. Not only were midwives prime targets of the Spanish Inquisition, old women were, too, particularly if they held their own property and were financially independent.[2]

It is a little-known fact that our U.S. Constitution is an almost exact copy of the Iroquois model of leadership (with which Thomas Jefferson was most impressed) but for one critical exception. We omitted the Grandmother Council, backbone of tribal decision-making. Imagine how different our society would be if the counsel of female elders was sought on all major environmental, economic, or political issues. Doubtless, the Grandmothers' advice would be in frequent opposition to male predilections for aggression, domination, and wastefulness, as well as the irrational justification of these.

Fortunately, there are some contemporary cultures that continue to hold elder women in high esteem. In Japan, a woman reaches the highest and most venerated stage of maturity at age sixty-one, an event always marked by ceremony. In certain Native-American- and South-American-Indian cultures, postmenopausal women acquire special status and privileges in the community as they transcend menstrual taboos. In China, too, elder woman are venerated and accorded respect.[3]

Beyond honor and veneration, elder women in early matrilineal cultures of the Middle East and Egypt performed many of society's most important and challenging roles. They dominated the healing arts, working as physicians, surgeons, and midwives. As scribes, they recorded for both temple and court, maintaining vital records and histories, setting up calendars and official tables of weights and measures, transcribing and editing scriptures, and running libraries. They were generally busier in their Crone years than in those of childbearing.[4] Mythology reiterates that the most critical inventions in the fields of medicine, nutrition, and food preparation were made by women in their "years of wisdom."

This last point raises an interesting question. How many years of wisdom did women actually have in these bygone eras? Isn't it true that until quite recently, the average life span for women was barely past menopause?

Interestingly, new evidence suggests that prehistoric women survived well past menopause. Anthropologists have struggled to make sense of this from an evolutionary standpoint: What was the point of women living far beyond their reproductive years? Based on their research of a tribe of modern-day hunter-gatherers known as the Hazda, Dr. Kristen Hawkes and colleagues believe that elder women of prehistory made an enormous, quantifiable difference to their kin. Among the Hazda, whenever a mother of young children has another baby and becomes absorbed with breast-feeding, it is only by intervention of an older female relative that the health of her other children are maintained:

> When a young woman [of the Hazda tribe] is burdened with a suckling infant and cannot fend for her family, she turns for support, not to her mate, but to a senior family relative—her mother, an aunt, an elder cousin. It is Grandma, or Grandma-proxy, who keeps the woman's other children in baobab and berries, Grandma who keeps them alive. She is not a sentiment; she is a requirement.[5]

On this basis, Hawkes and colleagues developed the Grandmother Hypothesis. They see the extension of life past menopause as a watershed event in prehistory. With elder women available to care for and secure food for the children, younger adults were free to roam and colonize new territories. Quite the opposite was true of primates whose juveniles had to feed themselves: They were confined to feeding grounds where the pickings were easy for young fingers. The presence of grandmothers allowed humans to migrate to places where securing food required full adult strength and cunning.[6]

Grandmother—surely this is the most powerful social role of woman throughout time. Even today, grandmothering makes all the difference to the child of a stressed and busy mother, as well as to the mother herself. The grandmother keeps the family together. Her nearly invisible role in our culture is one of real influence, in that attitudes, customs, ethical guidelines, and solutions to life's dilemmas are passed down through the matrilineal line.

Besides practical responsibilities, elder women of matrilineal cultures had metaphysical charges too. They facilitated most religious rites and official ceremonies, from birth to death. In terms of the afterlife, it was generally believed that one was taken up in the arms of the Mother, rather than, as by Christian tenets, to the bosom of the Father. In Buddhist and other Tantric traditions, three classes of priestess—*yogini, matri,* and *dakini*—represented the Virgin, Mother, and Crone. *Dakini* (the Crone) literally means "skywalker": Devoted to the destructive aspect, she prepared the dying, worked with bereaved families, and administered last rites. She also knew the way into the spirit realm and could be either fierce or gentle, depending on the dying one's behavior in life and lessons yet to be learned in crossing over.

Similarly, author Luisa Francia calls the Crone the "goddess of the crossroads" who can hinder or block one's way, kill or allow one to pass.[7] Tales and legends from all over the world teach that the path to knowledge or true love leads through an old woman: This witch (or woods-woman) appears so fragile or foolish that no one takes her seriously and then suddenly, she shows her power. In Greek myth, we know her as the trickster Hecate. In Syria, she is the huge-eyed goddess Mari, who searches men's souls. Her Christian adaptation is Aynat, the all-seeing Evil Eye. To a large extent, the ability to look through the veil that hides the future is the province of the Crone, although she may be blamed for events she has merely foretold.

Yet another mythic figure symbolizing the power of the Crone is Shakti, an amalgam of queenly strength, intelligence, grace, and sensuality. Across the board, Crone figures possess a strong sexual dimension, which clearly fits with the postmenopausal increase in testosterone. It's not the sensuality of the Crone that is frightening to men, but the combination of sexual power with emotional and intellectual autonomy (largely resulting from decreased estrogen/ progesterone).

Years ago, Rhonda L. Winn and Niles Newton did pivotal research on sexuality and aging in 106 indigenous cultures. In most of these, they found older women to be extremely interested in sex. In 22 percent of the cultures they studied, women became markedly less inhibited as they aged, displaying a wide range of sexually suggestive behaviors in public, from making copulatory movements while dancing to grabbing men's genitals or their own, often in a spirit of play. They also showed a great fondness for risqué jokes and anecdotes.[8] And in 70 percent of these societies (including the Loredu of South Africa, the Woges of New Guinea, and the Trobriand and Eastern Islanders), older women frequently had much younger men as sexual partners. Even very old women described by observers as "toothless and decrepit" were able to obtain young and attractive boys as lovers. Often, older women played the role of sexual initiator and instructor.

Why does this occur? Apart from soaring testosterone levels, this open sexuality is a natural expression of power in cultures in which older women maintain dominant social roles. In societies that disregard or frown on sexual activity among the aged, younger individuals tend to view their elders as undesirable or even repulsive.[9]

Until quite recently, this has been the case in the United States. According to a Consumers' Union survey conducted in 1989, 4,296 older respondents concurred that society considered them nonsexual. Only 65 percent of women over seventy were sexually active: A number had outlived their husbands and felt unprepared for the challenge of finding new partners or were confounded by the threat of sexually transmitted infection.[10] But now, as the baby boomers age, their characteristic pursuit of self-fulfillment has led to more enduring sexual expression (literally—thanks to Viagra).

Sexual expression among older women remains more acceptable in those who are married than in those who are single: We have a long way to go before our natural inclinations at this point in life are socially condoned. But couples, especially those who have been together for some time, have their own challenges. Rosalie Gilford, sociologist, sums it up this way: "Never in history have the lives of husbands and wives remained interwoven in intact marriages so long as to encounter the constellation of life-changing events that the last stages of the marital career now bring."[11] Unsettling differences may emerge at this point, especially if the couple has organized itself primarily around child rearing. And too, the hormonally induced role reversal continues to intensify with aging. But if partners are able to embrace these changes by giving each other space, a more androgynous companionship may ensue.

In bed, interesting possibilities develop. Viagra aside, men's slower arousal time and women's increased aggressiveness can lead to extended, even ritualistic lovemaking, with women in the lead. As Charlotte reports:

James and I have been together for forty-three years. We have four grown children and seven grandchildren. I suppose our sex life in the early years was like most others: James came quickly, was a little lacking in touch and timing, and my orgasms were sporadic at best. But I always loved to masturbate, and now, with the standards changing as they are, I find I can talk to him about the intimate details of my body. At first, I think I talked to cover his embarrassment at slowing down, complimenting him and teaching him at the same time, you might say. But oh, the times we have now…it's hours of pleasure for both of us!

Angelina has a different sort of story:

After I went through "the change" I felt different…drier, sometimes, and quite unsure of myself. But I wasn't the only one. Robert took longer to come around, and wanted to spend more time touching than ever before. At first, we were rather confused by all this, but eventually, our affection and companionship deepened, and we felt more alike, more in harmony with one another.

From Suzanne:

The best thing about sex after menopause is not caring anymore… sex no longer preoccupies your mind, your time, your body; you're not a victim of your drives. But when you get to it, it's just as good as ever, or even better. Maybe it's more like sex becomes part of everything else in your life. I honestly felt when menopause ended that I was no longer down in the dregs of my hormones, I was above it all, I had this overview all the time, and sex is thoroughly mixed into that.

And from Jeanne:

I'm almost seventy now, but I can't say that I feel old. Oh, sometimes I have days when I take it a bit slower, but generally, I feel vigorous and self-possessed. I've had my career, and children of whom I'm exceedingly proud—grandchildren, too!

Menopause was upsetting for me because my life was so hectic then, and I think my marriage suffered. But a few years later, something came over me and I felt this strength and confidence in myself, which reached full bloom in the bedroom. I had always liked sex and had orgasms easily, but now, there was another dimension. I'd lift off in my own thoughts and imagination, feeling a shift in consciousness almost on a regular basis. You know how it is when you're swept away by a really great orgasm, no idea how

you got there? Well, now I seemed to have ready access to those
places—freedom to fly, I called it. Really, this was quite the oppo-
site of what I expected sex to be like at this time of my life!

This account ties directly back to the power and authority of the
Crone, and, using Jeanne's terminology, it raises the crucial question: How can we realize the fullness of Cronehood and find the
freedom to fly, to traverse the higher realms with ease and confidence?

One way is to act on our natural authority at this stage and employ our wisdom. According to the Native-American "law of good
relationship," the Grandmother Council had the final say in setting
right any social or political misdeeds. For example, if a chief was
not leading his tribe in such a way that the people had adequate
food, water, and shelter, the Grandmothers had him replaced. Or
if in times of war, a chief instigated animosity to an extent that the
tribe's well-being was threatened, the Grandmothers would redirect
him or have him removed. Today, as women's groups increasingly
rally around issues of health care, the environment, education, gun
control, and violence, older women need to assume their natural
role of leadership. In this vein, Kitzinger describes postmenopausal
women in peasant societies of China and Spain as "political dyna-
mos, wheeling and dealing, plotting and scheming."[12]

Another way to take on added responsibility is to make room
for it. Loss of children from the home, loss of one's parents, and ultimately, loss of interest in maintaining "the nest" may lead the older
woman to weed out her possessions and pare her life down to the
essentials. Although this nest-dismantling behavior is often miscast
as symptomatic of "postmenopausal depression," it is really quite
common. Walking away from former entanglements for a simpler
way of life makes sense for women at this time.

Here is another gem of wisdom gleaned from the Menopause
Council: When I asked how I might increase my visionary experience, they advised me to (1) do less, and: (2) be unafraid to hold

the big space, especially if it looks like there's nothing in it. Thus, in keeping with the idea of role reversal at menopause, a woman who has played an active role in the world might choose to retreat, to travel on her own, or to relocate to a smaller and more suitable nest. Whatever we choose, the need for radical departure from obligatory roles as a means of finding deep intimacy with all of life is the key. It is within this framework that sexual fulfillment may be realized, if we so desire.

◎

CHAPTER 9

Healing *from* Abuse, Trauma, *and* Loss

Why a chapter on abuse in a book about sexual rhythms? Because most of us have experienced some form of violation, whether emotional, physical, sexual, gynecological, or obstetrical, that has negatively affected our intimate relationships. Sexual dysfunction occurs when we have lost the ability to be sexually self-determined and so have more or less sexual activity than suits us, whether by denial, inhibition, or compulsion.

We touched only briefly on abuse issues in Chapter 4, in terms of the potential of pregnancy to trigger memories of injuries long forgotten. It is estimated that at least one in four women have been sexually abused, and many do not remember it. How do we dredge from the depths what lies buried? How do we remember abuse?

Workshops on the subject are now widely available. Women who attend may think they are doing so out of simple curiosity until some long-repressed incident comes suddenly into focus. Skeptics say these workshops encourage women to fabricate memories by a process of group hypnosis or induced trance. Nonetheless, there is growing acknowledgment of the prevalence and devastating effects of abuse on our health, self-esteem, and the ability to form and sustain healthy relationships. At least women are now encouraged

187

to acknowledge a history of abuse rather than ignore it, as was previously expected.

Sexual Abuse

◎

A slow but undeniable shift is under way in cultural attitudes regarding abuse. Until quite recently, our criminal justice system showed great reluctance to prosecute abusers, particularly on the basis of children's testimony. Throughout the world, the belief that females are somehow responsible for their own abuse is deeply ingrained. Jurors may still decide that if a girl over the age of seven or so is abused, it may be because she has behaved or dressed seductively. Women who are raped often face similar assumptions; they may be grilled as to what they were wearing or how they were behaving when the crime occurred. Thus it is hardly surprising that rape is underreported: A 2007 government report in England estimated that between 75 and 95 percent of rape crimes are never reported to the police.[1]

Although rape is underreported, we know that it happens to a woman once every two minutes in the United States, and once every seventeen seconds in South Africa.[2] As much as possible, we must take measures to protect ourselves: We must avoid situations that might jeopardize us. In the end, even when a case goes to trial and a woman is vindicated, she usually bears scars of her violation that are very difficult to heal.

Date rape is in a class by itself. When a woman is raped by someone she agreed to go out with, she may feel guilty and repress the incident. The same is true for the woman raped by her partner or spouse. Here are some questions to help you assess whether you might be a victim: Have you ever been made to have sex against your will? Have you ever been forcibly restrained or held down for sex while clearly indicating you wanted to be free? If so, you have indeed been raped.

Questions used to unearth sexual abuse by an acquaintance or relative are a bit subtler. Have you ever been tricked into an intimate situation you did not desire? Has anyone ever touched you intimately against your will? Do you have a lot of trouble surrendering during lovemaking? Do you hate being touched? Do you have trouble setting boundaries with others? Do you find great difficulty in trusting others, especially members of the opposite sex? Do you continually find yourself stuck in relationships? Do you suffer from chronic illness, particularly gynecological problems? Do you often feel outside yourself when you have sex? If these questions trigger even an inkling of response, contact a support organization and get help.

Sometimes, memories of abuse are triggered by stressful situations or life-changing events such as divorce, loss of home or income, natural disaster, death of a loved one, serious physical injury to oneself or a loved one, or physical violence of any kind. In short, anything that causes us to feel pushed to our limits and vulnerable is apt to release the subconscious and bring unpleasant memories to the surface.

This woman's story serves to illustrate:

We were making love and were hot into it. My husband pushed me over on my side to enter me from behind, which I really didn't want, and suddenly, something just went off inside me and I panicked. Not in my head but in my heart, my gut, I felt this constriction, this fear. I knew it had nothing to do with him, but I couldn't deny the feeling. Actually, I had noticed this before in other situations with men when I felt they were manipulating me. I noticed the same fear and this feeling of terror, just below the surface. Part of me would freeze up and go limp, as if in survival mode.

Finally, through hypnosis, I remembered some friend of my uncle's forcing me to let him play with my nipples, show him my backside and let him finger me, just a little on the outside. That's all that ever happened, but I responded in that same way back then—I froze, stood still, felt very much in danger but powerless to cry out. I felt totally humiliated, like I was no good, dirty, and it was my fault.

Once I got over this, I could see what was happening with my husband. Whenever he was forceful with me, even if it was really okay, I just froze up—I couldn't help it. And if I let him go ahead anyway, I had those same feelings of self-loathing. We had some stuff to work out, I can tell you!

In a moment, we will look further at how abuse affects sexuality. But first, here are some additional characteristics and modes of behavior common in women who have been abused.

- describes self as never having been a child
- extremely concerned with control
- overly willing to expose genitals to others
- unexplained pain with intercourse
- extreme ideas about sexuality
- hypersensitive to touch
- repeatedly exploited by others in relationship
- deeply estranged from family
- general feeling of being "under it"
- detaches from self and others
- nothing ever wrong with life, always neutral
- childlike behavior, dress, or appearance
- unkempt personal appearance
- chaotic surroundings and habits
- overly controlled surroundings or habits
- no personal boundaries
- no trust
- anger inappropriate or out of proportion to the situation
- inability to appreciate others
- blind adoration of others

○ fanatic religious or philosophical beliefs

○ jumps into situations and to conclusions

○ difficulty with decision making[3]

From this list, it is easy to extrapolate sexual response patterns of abusees, which range from total shutdown to compulsive sexual activity and display. The latter may be surprising, but it is as if the victim were saying, "See, I'm so sexual and out there with it that no one can take control of me—I'm in charge." This attitude generally precludes the surrender that leads to orgasm, and it almost certainly precludes intimacy. It bespeaks the stereotypical male approach to sex, that of using sex primarily for self-gratification and without the context of relationship. Women who have been abused may thus unconsciously reject their feminine vulnerability to be more on a par with their oppressor. Clarisse related, "In retrospect, it's like I bought into the beliefs of the man who abused me. My cunt was just a cunt, and I used it that way, keeping myself separate from it, using it as much as I could to prove the point that it was not me, I didn't have to be connected."

The psychological effects of abuse that increase vulnerability to disease, accidents, and other calamities are more difficult to track. Many characteristics of abusees are in fact contradictory, though decidedly extreme. Bipolar personality disorder often correlates to a history of sexual abuse.

Besides rape and sexual abuse, women may be abused in intimate health-care situations. Have you ever felt violated during a gynecological exam; for example, by procedures or tools used forcibly to examine you when you clearly were not ready? Or, if you have given birth, did you feel abused by procedures or technology used without your full consent and understanding? These types of abuse may be less obvious because they are part of the cultural milieu, but the effects are the same: self-esteem and self-worth are diminished, personal boundaries are lost or disrupted, and sexual response and satisfaction are reduced.

In my many years of practicing women's health care, I have had ample experience with women suffering from what is commonly known as vaginismus, or the uncontrollable contraction of vaginal muscles if penetration is attempted. Typically caused by an unnecessarily rough initial gynecological exam, it is especially sad to see in very young women who may find it almost impossible to have intercourse, let alone regular checkups. Of course, vaginismus is also a classic sign of sexual abuse.

When working with a woman who has this problem, I go out of my way to put her in control. I suggest the use of a small speculum, and I teach her how to insert it herself. Sometimes this is not possible, and we need to stop, take a moment, then start again by having her put a finger inside to feel how her muscles contract so that she can work directly on relaxing them. This alone will not cure her condition; the same involuntary response will probably occur the next time she agrees to penetration. But at least she may gain the self-confidence to seek help, work on herself, and communicate her needs and fears to her partner.

If she cannot come to terms with her situation, she may find that the only way she can have sex is by disassociation. This is tragic because the pattern perpetuates itself, and the woman remains a victim.

Classic therapeutic techniques for vaginismus include behavioral approaches. The woman is asked to relax thoroughly and then imagine, step-by-step, the stages of intercourse while trying to stay open as much as possible. Sometimes plastic dilators are used by the woman to simulate penetration by another in conjunction with visualization.[4] The trouble with this approach is that it may not allow the necessary release of emotion, particularly of anger. And penetration is not the be-all and end-all of sexual pleasure for women that it is for men.

In my opinion, the best remedy for women struggling with vaginismus is a body-based therapy, such as hypnotherapy or Eye Movement Desensitization Reprocessing (EMDR), which accesses the subconscious to allow emotional release in a controlled environment. Northrup concurs: "Lower chakra [sexual] wounds don't heal until they're witnessed."[5]

At the same time, if the woman is partnered, she can talk to him or her and forge an exploration agreement. That is, they agree to let her take the lead in showing all the finer points of what is arousing to her; what particularly gives her pleasure. She can begin by demonstrating what she does when she masturbates, exactly where and how she likes to be touched. Then she can guide her partner to try the same, if she likes, but with the understanding that they will go no further on that occasion. She must always be in control and in charge of the pace, doing as much or as little as seems right to her, with her right to stop the process at any time fully understood.

In a similar vein is the trauma attendant to an unplanned or undesired episiotomy. As discussed in Chapter 5, there are practical considerations in healing the vaginal area when there has been injury, and most women who have had repair have a certain amount of hesitation the first time they have sex again. But some feel more than hesitation: They feel violated, mutilated, no longer themselves. The psychological trauma of episiotomy is similar to that of sexual abuse in that the sufferer may feel shame, guilt, anger, or inadequacy.

The healing process for any type of abuse must incorporate factual information, enough to help a woman see her trauma in the larger social context so she realizes that she is not the only one to whom this violation has occurred. Ultimately, she needs support in releasing the power her wounds have held over her life. This seldom takes place overnight.

Physical Abuse

◎

Many of the impacts of sexual abuse occur in women who have experienced physical abuse. If this is your current situation, you should be aware of the rules governing health-care providers as regards visible signs or a claim of abuse; in most states, we are mandated to report the situation to family services (a division of social services). The perpetrator may then be arrested but if able to post bail, he or she may be released without warning unless state or county rules require it.

If you are being physically abused, you must get help, as your perpetrator will not stop without treatment (even though he or she may swear never to do it again), and your life is in jeopardy. Contact a domestic-violence hotline: They will let you know your rights and advise you on staying safe if arrest occurs.

As with sexual abuse, body-based therapy with expert facilitation is the best option for treatment. You may be surprised to learn that physical abuse/domestic violence crosses all socio-economic boundaries, and that women who stay in abusive relationships do so for a variety of reasons, not the least of which is financial concern for themselves and/or their children. As with any trauma, hypervigilance (permanent red-alert state) may result, which is quite the opposite of the receptivity needed for sexual fulfillment.

Emotional Abuse

◎

Whatever happens to a woman's body also happens to her spirit. Thus emotional abuse is an undeniable component of physical abuse. When a woman is raped, she suffers much more than physical injury. Feelings of terror and utter powerlessness combined with the threats or insults of her attacker have as far-reaching effects as does the degradation of her body. The same is true for victims of domestic violence. Girls who are victims of incest likewise feel the psychological manipulations of a trusted relative to be just as devastating as the physical violation.

But emotional abuse may also stand alone, often manifesting in destructive relationships that tend to be repeated. Since both sexes are susceptible to the emotional manipulations of others, we must look beyond misogyny for causes.

We can trace some of our susceptibility to emotional abuse to early childhood experience, particularly as regards attachment to our parents. Avodah Offit, author of *The Sexual Self,* says sexual behavior is very much influenced by the degree to which we have bonded to our mother (or other loving adult) in infancy, as this directly affects how we tolerate separation anxiety. If we are kept close and secure when young, we are comfortable with ourselves as we mature and are better able to handle being alone. If, as asserted by philosopher and psychologist William James, "The greatest terror of infancy is solitude," perhaps we must reassess our ways of fostering independence in our young. Putting our children on their own at an early age has been a survival strategy in a culture moving too fast for intimate relationship; it really has not worked for them or for us. The more healthy and sound our early attachments, the less susceptible we are to unhealthy, compulsive/abusive relationships.

A great turning point and reckoning in this regard occurs when we first fall in love. Separation anxiety becomes intense as we realize that in bonding and attaching deeply to another, our bonds to our parents will be forever changed. Our need to be close, to be protected and to protect, are suddenly transferred to someone new.

Ideally, this separation anxiety and the concomitant desire for closeness motivate us to endure the challenging stages of intimate relationship. It might well be said that strong bonds in infancy are the only basis for meeting life's onslaughts with courage and equanimity. If these original attachments are impaired, things predictably go awry as subsequent attachments are apt to be inhibited or fragmented. The less we are able to connect with and trust others, the greater our anxiety and dependence. Thus we become ready targets for emotional abuse.

And yet, even with sound initial attachments, we are so vulnerable when we first fall in love that reimprinting may occur.

Psychologist Albert Ellis believes that dysfunctional patterns in a relationship can be traced to our first sexual interaction. Here are some questions to help you evaluate your own experience: Did your first love share his/her heart with you, or just his/her body? Was he/she patient and kind, or uncaring and inconsiderate? Was he/she honest and forthright with you, or deceiving and untrue? Did the relationship end amicably or with unresolved anger, pain, and humiliation? Did you feel in any way abused by him/her?

We may thus define emotional abuse as any behavior that subjugates us through intimidation, ridicule, invalidation, manipulation, or verbal assault. Check out this list of indicators cited by Mickey Sperlich and Julia Seng in their book, *Survivor Moms,* to see if any fit your experience. You can identify emotional abuse if your partner has ever:

- consistently ignored your feelings
- ridiculed or insulted women as a group
- insulted your valued beliefs, religion, race, heritage, or class
- withheld approval or affection as punishment
- criticized you or called you names
- insulted your family or friends
- humiliated you
- repeatedly refused to socialize with you
- kept you from working, controlled your money, made all decisions
- refused to work or share money
- taken your car keys or money away
- regularly threatened to leave or told you to leave
- punished the children when angry at you
- threatened to hurt you or your family
- threatened to take the children if you left
- abused pets to hurt you
- manipulated you with lies and contradictions[6]

Sometimes it's easier to recognize the effects of emotional abuse than the contributing behavior. If you suffer from low self-esteem, mistrust of your perceptions, an inability to appreciate your accomplishments, a lack of motivation, chronic depression, or difficulty in taking charge of your life, you are probably a victim.

Emotional abuse may also occur in sexual encounters: I've worked with women, otherwise confident and secure, who have been devastated by a partner's assessment that their vagina was too loose, too tight, too long, or too short, that their sexual intensity was not up to par, or that their nipples were not pink enough, large enough, hard enough, and so on. I am both frustrated and saddened by the frequency with which women question the adequacy of their bodies, the appearance of breasts and genitals that are perfectly normal. It is important to remember that sexual domination victimizes us as surely as more direct forms of abuse.

As is clear from the above list, it is also crucial that we not minimize the effects of coercion, another common strategy of emotional abusers. Whenever an intimate partner makes us feel inadequate, or tries to place the responsibility for his or her happiness on us, we are looking at emotional abuse.

Five Profiles of Abusees

◎

In *The Emotionally Abused Woman*, Beverly Engel presents five distinct profiles of chronic abusees, each of which finds a complement in a particular type of abuser. Abusers can be anyone in a role of authority: parents, teachers, bosses, mentors, or religious leaders. They may also be peer counterparts such as siblings, co-workers, friends, or lovers.[7]

Note that these abuser/abusee configurations have no rank of superiority or inferiority. But all too often, women move from one configuration to another. The main thing abusee roles have in common is that they align with feelings of powerlessness and inadequacy. Women predisposed to being abused are apt to step into one of these roles just as they begin to care deeply for another; for it is precisely at this point that their deep conditioning is triggered.

Here, then, are five profiles of abusees. Although there are similarities among these types, there are subtle differences in the sort of partner each type tends to select.

Selfless and Silent

The selfless and silent woman has usually been dominated, controlled, or neglected in her youth to such an extreme that she has little sense of self. She may take on the personality of others, particularly in love—anything to be accepted. On the other hand, intimacy may feel frightening and threatening to her.

When it comes to sex, she moves in and out of relationships with great frequency. Sex may be deeply inhibited or explosive as it releases deep emotions that cannot be integrated. Women in this role are in turmoil when in love, empty when not. As one of my clients confided to me:

> I don't really know how to be close to a man, but I sure do try. Usually I try to be like him, doing what he likes to do, even in bed, no matter what. Sometimes I feel hurt, used, and very sad, and then I get so pissed off and furious I have to leave. I hate that, though, because when I'm by myself I feel so empty. That scares me so much I start looking for someone else right away.

Under these circumstances, intimacy is elusive. As Offit observes, "In bed, dependence more often leads to erotic extinction than to an eternal flame of passion."[8] Women of selfless temperament are usually attracted to their opposite: a narcissistic type with little ability to care for another. The longer they stay with a partner like this, the more they are apt to be drawn into his or her grandiose schemes. If and when they decide to leave, they will have to cope with the loss of all they have invested, plus a further diminished sense of self.

Women thus afflicted need professional help to trace patterns of self-abuse back to their original source.

Servile and Compulsive

Women in the servile and compulsive role are centered on the expectations of others. Almost every woman today has some "pleaser" in her, so deeply ingrained is the expectation that we put others' needs before our own. But the servile/compulsive woman takes this to an extreme; she will tolerate and suffer the demeaning and abusive behavior of others to an extent that is damaging to all concerned. Just as she blames herself for the misdeeds of her intimates, she likewise impedes them from taking responsibility for their actions. If she happens on a moment of clarity and notices how others take advantage of her, she usually apologizes for her behavior, repressing herself and remaining dependent.

Why does a woman behave thus? Typically, her parents ignored her personal boundaries. Thus she evaluates her behavior as performance, assessing it by her partner's standards. "Was it good enough?" she queries, "Was I okay, are you sure it was really all right?" Unlike the selfless/silent type, she rarely knows the benefits of explosive release. She is in a constant quandary as regards her adequacy—preoccupied, distracted from herself, and intent on measuring up. Or she may avoid sex altogether, focusing her anxiety on her career, her children's accomplishments, the cleanliness of her house, and so on. In short, she is mortally afraid of losing control, and of letting the monster of her own frustrated needs and desires out of the bag.

Typically, she does not reach orgasm with intercourse. There are many reasons a woman might not have an orgasm, but in this case, the servile/compulsive woman cannot connect with herself enough to let go. For her, the *petite morte* of orgasm is downright terrifying. As Karen related:

I try to give my lover everything she wants in bed—I give and give until honestly, I feel weak and sick inside. Nothing I do seems to really excite her, and when she finally comes, I start worrying about what she's thinking and whether or not I've really pleased her. I know I shouldn't say this, but I'd rather put my energy into the house or my work, where I know I can do some good.

Sadly, this woman is often paired with a controlling type, one who continually reinforces her need to please by being hypercritical of her.

The servile/compulsive woman needs to learn that life is not about meeting an outside standard of perfection but about loving and developing herself. She must practice putting herself first, letting go, and having fun (it won't come naturally). This often involves attaching some name or face from the past to the censoring voice of her inner critic. Her key to happiness is reconnecting with her wild, original self, then getting back on her own track in life. Sexually, she will need a new foundation based on her own needs and desires. She may need professional help with this.

Guilt-Ridden and Reactive

The guilt-ridden and reactive role is that of the sinner. The woman playing it is more physically expressive than other types we've discussed, but her passions bring only guilt and shame. She is so burdened with self-loathing that she barely relates to her partner, and sex holds no intimacy for her. Women in this role are often victims of physical or severe emotional abuse, taught to believe their inherent naughtiness, seductiveness, or worthlessness are just cause for violation. As adults, they are in reaction to these imprints. Engel puts it most succinctly: "Sinners believe that bad things only happen to bad people."[9]

Guilt-ridden/reactive women typically choose partners who reinforce their guilt by blaming them for everything under the sun, which only perpetuates their feelings of unworthiness. Blamers are typically passionate but reactive, unrealistic and unstable, and are likely to be closet sinners. But whoever plays the role of blamer is always right: the sinner, always wrong.

As Sharon revealed:

My boyfriend says terrible things to me sometimes, and I know I should forgive him but I just can't. Then I see even more how he's right—I really am a terrible person. I don't do the shopping on time because I want to read instead, or I forget to pay bills because I'm out with my friends.

What about her sex life?

I really like sex, but I get scared and nervous about it. If I mess up, I cry and have to stop, I feel so awful inside, and he tells me it's my fault. He's right, of course, but that just makes it worse. Sometimes I go out with other guys and it's better, but I'm scared that my boyfriend will find out. The truth is, I like sex, but I hate what it does to me.

The guilt-ridden/reactive woman absorbs her partner's ills and delusions without discrimination. Their relationship is so volatile and out of balance that she rightly equates love with pain. She must learn to distinguish positive, life-affirming passions from negative, destructive ones and start listening to her own voice, seeing her worth apart from the opinions of others. This means ridding herself of shadows, those of blamers past and present. Frequently, there is a history of alcoholism or drug abuse in the family, and she, her partner, or both are dependent. Professional help is once again in order.

Passive and Victimized

Women in a passive role are targets for victimization. Sexually, they are easily manipulated and apt to be used, perpetually finding themselves in the wrong place at the wrong time with the wrong person. The victim's life is ridden with anxiety and highly affected by the maneuvers of others. Frequently, she partners with those who dis-empower her by invalidating her actions and perceptions. The more she is invalidated, the greater her passivity and dependence.

Since her intimate partners have full sway, she accepts their ver-bal or physical abuse. The victim tells herself she deserves it because she's inept or crazy. Most likely, she experienced a similar pattern at home.

This woman's partner may be a bit of a sociopath, living for con-quest without any hint of regard for her. Typically, the sociopath is largely admired (except by those who have seen through the facade). Deviously and methodically, he or she manipulates this woman into submission by not responding to her advances but insisting that she be responsive. He or she bestows affection only when she is extremely busy, and then accuses her of being cold when she is not ready. He or she may make her question her sanity by pretending never to have said or done things that were quite de-liberate: In other words, he or she is a master at making others feel uncomfortable while seeming to do nothing at all.[10]

With sociopaths, sex goes only one way: their own. They are completely in charge, calling all the shots. The victim will feel igno-rant and inadequate, convinced there is something seriously wrong with her sexual ability. As Julie says:

> *The only time sex was any good for me was when we were making up—it gave me a chance to express my love to Gene, to reassure myself that he still loved me. The rest of the time I felt too insecure to make any moves in bed, and I don't think Gene wanted me to anyway—I had so many problems. Sometimes, though, I let him force me into it. I suffered through, hoping I could improve myself in his eyes.*

Passive victim types may be helped with support groups. Coun-seling is crucial, and social support, including legal assistance, is es-sential if physical violence has occurred.

Hysterical and Overdrawn

The hysterical and overdrawn woman is the last type we will consider. The word *hysterical* derives from the Latin word for "uterus," and common use of the term harks back to a time when irrational or highly excitable women were believed to be under the influence of uterine "ethers" moving about their body. The somewhat less derogatory term *histrionic* is now more commonly used. I rather like the term *hysterical* because it implies a woman under the influence of feminine energies and forces, albeit to an extreme.

Women thus oriented thrive on chaos, high drama, and intensity. From an early age they were either strictly controlled and inhibited or wracked with constant crisis and disruption. Either way, they feel most alive and comfortable in the midst of (or while making) a scene. They consistently seek situations that engender strong emotions like anger or jealousy: anything to stir things up a bit. They often choose unstable partners in unstable circumstances. There is a strong tendency to upset the balance continually, or to become involved in confrontations that are irreconcilable.

When it comes to love and sex, a woman of this kind will generally choose unwisely, perhaps a severely antisocial partner or a near psychopath. She may be attracted to a substance abuser, compulsive gambler, a sex addict, or someone in trouble with the law. She may go for the "hard cases," individuals so disturbed that they are nearly impossible to reach. She may also choose someone unavailable (married, for example) or clearly not interested. She is not apt to select a healthy, somewhat normal person with a decent likelihood of loving her and treating her respectfully.

The hysterical and overdrawn woman uses drama as a smoke screen to avoid looking at her problems. Her partner is doing the same; it is the main thing they have in common. Tension is her drug, and she uses it to keep chaos at a level that feels familiar and comfortable. Setting ultimatums, staging rescues and arguments, she makes her partner's problems her own, creating so much stress in their relationship that abuse may come as a welcome release.

Sexually, it's a roller coaster. This woman's counterpart usually has a highly volatile personality, which may be further intensified by drugs, alcohol, intrigue, or criminal activity. Sex can be unbelievably hot and explosive, at the same time riddled with cruelty and manipulation. The most noticeably absent quality in both partners is genuine vulnerability.

Here's a typical report:

> *The best thing about our relationship was the sex. I loved to entice Jack into sex when he wasn't really in the mood. Sometimes I'd have to make a scene, accuse and argue with him just to get him angry and really hot for me. Then he'd take me to the limit, and I'd scream and holler my way to oblivion. Other times he was cold, cruel, and calculating. If I let him make love to me like that, he would trick me out—you know, make it hard for me to come, or make me come when I wasn't ready. I'd be so angry that I'd pull way back. Then he would apologize, and we'd have blowout sex again.*

Note the contradictions here: On the one hand, sex was "the best thing"; on the other hand, it was degrading. Clearly, this woman must learn to find stability and security within herself. She must learn to use her lust for excitement in constructive ways, or she is destined for serious burnout. To do this, she needs a counselor's help. Even if not drug or alcohol dependent herself, she may benefit from contact with an abusers' or a family of alcoholics' group, exploring the characteristics of relationship under the shadow of dependency.

◎   ◎   ◎

If we are honest with ourselves, we will all admit that we have played at least one of these roles to some extent in our lives. Whether we have experienced emotional, sexual, or physical abuse, the bottom line is the same: We must acknowledge and effectively address it.

However, we must also give ourselves permission to work sensitively on these issues. Any woman who has been forced or compelled into intimate contact against her best interests must feel free to follow her instincts in this regard. Healing work is rhythmic: two steps forward, one step back, rather like birthing a baby. If we push it, we may sink back into feelings of powerlessness and inertia.

Sexual Addiction

◎

Let us not confuse sexual addiction with a healthy appetite for intimacy! Some women want and have sex several times a day, especially in the early stages of relationship. When we fall in love, most of us long for our partners so much that we can hardly endure physical separation. This is not an addiction, but bonding, healthy attachment behavior.

Despite this, there is some evidence that women may not be as monogamous by nature as previously thought. Biologically, the fact that male sperm are not merely egg-seeking but have block and attack mechanisms against alien sperm suggests an adaptation made to females with more than one partner.[11] In earlier eras, frequent childbearing and extended breast-feeding rendered women anovulatory for long enough periods that they could easily be with a number of partners without consequence of pregnancy. This was particularly true of hunter-gatherer women, reportedly so active that they rarely ovulated.[12]

Unlike most modern societies that still fall prey to the Madonna/Whore dichotomy, there were numerous pre-Christian traditions that honored women who were sexually wise. These women were the sexual initiators of young men, in the tradition of the vestal virgins of ancient Greece, or the sacred *dakinis* of the East. Figures of sexually empowered women carved or cast long ago can still be found today, displaying their genitals or opening them to view, like

Kali of India or Sheila-Na-Gig of Celtic traditions.[13] Women who find that they impart profound wisdom though sexual contact, especially if the experience feels sacred and happens to them repeatedly, are likely to have an active sexual history that is far from promiscuous.

However, if sex is a drug used to avoid difficulties in life or to find validation that should come from inside, this is a problem. It's a fine line: We all use sex occasionally for reassurance or to meet our most basic needs for intimate contact. But when sexual activity undermines our work or professional relationships, or when it is hurtful to others, sexuality is no longer in its proper life-affirming place.

Consider this case history of a woman caught in compulsive sexual behavior. Tina reported a tempestuous and stressful phase in a career she wanted to escape: She was overworked and completely exhausted. She met up with an old friend, now married, and despite her better judgment, started sleeping with him. In her words:

It's not like we were in love. I felt comfortable with him, and it was a fantastic release. But the more we did it, the less I felt. I don't know how to describe it; it was like I was numb, emotionally dead inside. Still, he took good care of me, got me nice things, all that....

Then, of all things, I got pregnant! I'd only been pregnant once before and this was a complete accident, total carelessness. It shocked me into seeing what I was doing...I wasn't taking care of myself at all, I was just using sex to get by. So I had an abortion and ended the relationship.

Tina represents the otherwise assertive woman who becomes a passive victim in relationship. Work-related stress, uncertainty about the future, and inability to deal with impending changes in life can lead to self-destructive behavior.

Another example from Janelle, married with a child:

My husband was the classic executive, straight arrow, in his head and anxious all the time. After our son was born, sex just stopped. I felt dried up inside, like I was losing my beauty and my charm.

I started an affair with a man in the neighborhood—he was un-employed and his wife worked—I even knew her slightly. He had problems, and I tried to help. It was so wonderful to be needed and to be admired, to have that hot kind of sex that is just so good! But after a while I started seeing him for what he was: a loser, pure and simple, and somebody else's husband. Quite suddenly I saw that I'd been using him to avoid the disappointment I felt in my own marriage, and my anxiety about finding a life of my own. It was a rude awakening to have to look at things I'd been putting off for a long time.

Examples like this are common enough. Then again, sexual addiction may link to an insatiable sexual appetite: a condition we call nymphomania. Sex therapists concur that nymphomania results from a lack of healthy attachment and separation when young. Nymphomaniacs can't bear to be alone; they desperately crave the comforts of human contact, presumably to compensate for some deprivation experienced in childhood.

Women who consistently bed new partners, who are always "on the make," typically have such high anxiety that sex, no matter how frequent, doesn't make a dent in their insecurity. Although some are orgasmic, most report orgasms as unfulfilling and monotonous, with the vast majority being rarely orgasmic. The out-of-control aspect of the nymphomaniac's behavior makes it difficult for her to let go. In short, nymphomaniacs are, for the most part, profoundly immature, deeply injured, and repressed.

The Impact of Loss

◎

Personal traumas are also likely to interfere with a woman's sex life, particularly the loss of a loved one. The death of a child, parent, other relative, or a dear friend may cause a desperate need for contact or complete disinterest. If only one partner is affected, the other may provide stable ground. But if both are devastated, the emotional intensity of sex may be just too much to handle. Rhythms of processing grief are often at odds: When one partner is raw and vulnerable, the other is shut down and unable to feel much of anything. Here is Amanda's story of what happened to her after the death of her son at eight weeks from SIDS (sudden infant death syndrome):

> *I don't think there is anything more horribly painful on earth than losing a child—at least, I hope there's not, because I don't think I could endure it. Jerry and I had many sad and upsetting experiences trying to make love after Jason's death, but this one time was so amazing I must share it with you. We were fucking and crying, really, fucking and crying, when we felt something descend on us, a deep break in the tension, a feeling of warmth and healing. It was so wonderful, I can't tell you…like we were in a perfect state of grace. Sex aside, orgasm aside, in that moment, time stood still and we were okay again. After this, we stopped doubting and blaming ourselves so much. The guilt began to lift, and we began to live day by day.*

Reestablishing intimacy after any kind of intensely painful loss is a difficult process; this couple was lucky to find common ground. Time heals, but the road is rocky and uneven. Realigning ourselves after sustaining trauma is hardly a simple matter; layer upon layer must be permeated with new hope and resolve. Once we encouraged survivors to express their grief profoundly and immediately, believing that if they did so, they would be over it; now we know that mourning is in fact a cyclical process and may extend for years and years, even a lifetime. The same is true, by the way, for anyone recovering from experiences of physical, emotional, or sexual abuse. Tina relates:

> *Pat and I had known each other for about a year, while she was still living with her former partner. Then she and I became intimate, and she decided to leave Sue. She felt a lot of guilt about this*

decision, along with sadness and confusion regarding her patterns of passivity from childhood abuse. Just as she became free to be with me, she decided she couldn't be sexual for a while. That was okay; I understood.

And what about trauma from abortion? This is, in my experience, virtually unaddressed in most cultures today. Carol Leonard, midwife and abortion counselor, has placed pink hearts along the hallway to the procedure room, featuring words from those who have already undergone abortion there. This is what they say:

I am twenty. I have a beautiful two-year-old daughter at home, but I'm still in school and living with my parents. I made this decision so my baby wouldn't be brought into a life I wasn't ready to give it. I believe that when I'm ready, this baby will be given back to me, when I can devote my life to him/her.

◎   ◎   ◎

When I found out I was pregnant, I had so many thoughts. I'm eighteen years old. I work three jobs, and I try very hard to be successful. I find having an abortion a very difficult decision, but I know it's right, despite a strong maternal instinct. With that instinct, I think about what my child's life would be like. I know what it's like to not be wanted. I never want my child to feel that way.

◎   ◎   ◎

Today is the hardest decision I've ever made in my life. There is nothing in this world I love more than children, but another one is not an option for me right now. My son is only seven months old. He is so young; it's just not fair to take his mother's time and love away from him. I am a single mom, and it is more than hard. Two infants are way too much for me! I make this decision for my son and for myself.

◎   ◎   ◎

Thank you for supporting my decision to have a second chance at being a young woman again. You have saved my life.

Unprocessed grief from abortion merits counseling. Check out online resources, such as *Exhale* (http://exhaleprovoice.org). Raise the subject with friends who may also benefit from help.

◎   ◎   ◎

If you have a history of any of the experiences discussed in this chapter, please see the "Women's Worksheet on Abuse and Trauma" in the Appendix. In addition to the topics we have covered, it addresses other events in life that can generate extreme stress. These are listed at the end of the worksheet, and although you are asked to rate their severity, there is no scoring system but your own. This worksheet is meant to prompt self-reflection and healing, but if you feel the need, get a therapist's help. Mickey Sperlich (whose work was pivotal to this worksheet's development) observes that more than three experiences of abuse or severe stress may result in post-traumatic stress disorder (PTSD). If you think you are at risk, definitely seek the assistance of a counselor familiar with this disorder.

For any woman with a history of abuse or trauma, one healing option is to forego sex until the ground is set for healthier patterns of intimacy. In the next chapter, we will look at celibacy as an increasingly common choice for women trying to heal from trauma or rid themselves of destructive sexual behaviors.

CHAPTER 10

Choosing Celibacy

Women who decide to abstain from sex, for whatever reason, have been looked upon as something of an anomaly. To be sexually active is so deeply ingrained in the usual definition of happiness that a woman without a partner is presumed to be longing and deprived. As we will see in the forthcoming pages, nothing could be further from the truth, at least when abstinence is a choice.

In fact, a growing number of women choose to take a break from sexual activity when personal problems or crises intervene. This coincides with great gains in women's social and economic autonomy. Cultural constraints that once put the reins of a woman's sexual activity in the hands of her male provider no longer hold sway. Women may still be viewed as sex objects, but increasingly are shown by the media to have sexual identities of their own. It is no longer unacceptable that women choose, particularly under circumstances of stress or trauma, to forego sex in order to conserve energy.

To illustrate, here is my own story. It was 1982, and my ex-husband and I were going through a particularly difficult time in our relationship; we were not yet married (a bone of contention between us) and were working out negative consequences of an affair he'd had at the beginning of our relationship. That these issues had disrupted our sex life seemed natural to me, although I won't deny I was concerned. Our therapist, a supposed expert in sexual dysfunction, somehow thought it necessary to show us a video of a couple engaged in foreplay, with step-by-step instructions. This experience both mortified and infuriated me, and I told her outright, "I don't need this, I don't think we have any problems with technique. My problem is with my feelings, my pain and vulnerability, the trust issue. If we work on these, maybe I'll want to have sex again."

This is not to minimize sex therapy for those with unusual aversions or compulsions, but for the vast majority of women, sexual dysfunction is emotionally based, nothing more. We don't need another survey to tell us that a woman cannot be loving, open, and orgasmic if she feels her partner is treating (or has treated) her poorly or unfairly, let alone if she feels she can't be heard.

What is it like to take a sexual time-out? It depends on the situation, but most women report initial loneliness and/or relief, followed by renewed self-confidence and clarity. Brenda, a single woman in her thirties, tells how a series of relationships frightened her into abstinence that then became voluntary for a period of seven months:

> I had an outrageous affair with a fellow who turned out to be royalty, a Scottish lord in fact. It was a whirlwind romance, and in a matter of weeks he proposed marriage. On the one hand, I knew I'd be taken care of for life, and all my friends were telling me to go for it. But this is a pattern that keeps repeating in my life—guys go crazy for me, and the situation becomes overwhelming. Maybe I have something to do with it—after all, I let it happen, to a point. Then I feel this pressure of being swept away, and I just pull back or quit. I do notice that it happens more when I'm unsettled or stressed at work.
>
> So, I said no to this guy with much relief; then the same thing happened with a man who turned out to be married—there were signs and signals that I never followed up until it was way too late. After this I pulled back completely from men and sex.

Being celibate all this time has given me some important things. One is protection—I can feel vulnerable with myself and not be at risk. Another is a very clear picture of what I want in relationship—marriage to the right man. Eventually, because now I'm content to wait.

Other comments from women in similar circumstances: "I'm pleased and proud to be nurturing *me*," "I see the seeds of myself beginning to grow," "I have inner conviction now—I'm my own person." Voluntary abstinence may thus be a rite of passage for women today, particularly in response to eased sexual mores.

Yet another factor in a woman's choice of celibacy is the desire to reconnect with her body and feel her own rhythms. In other cultures, women have had regular opportunity for a sexual time-out via isolation during menstruation. This not only allowed them to separate from men for a few days, but it also provided an opportunity to disentangle from routine obligations and reflect on personal issues. We all need such a respite, a chance to keep body and soul to ourselves periodically without guilt or anxiety. Without this, we may get stuck in patterns of self-denial and subservience.

As Lynda explains:

I grew up in a household where Mom's main task was taking care of everyone else's business. I loved her for it, hated her for it, and learned to depend on her and not myself. Even though we fought bitterly when I was in my teens, I found myself continually dependent and wanting to please her before myself. Three marriages and three children later, I still don't know all that much about me. My sexuality has been confined, I think, to what's been expected.

I've been abstinent for three months now, and it's been a good way for me to sort things out and get to the heart of who I am. To tell you the truth, I feel like a kid again, discovering broken threads from the past and reweaving them. Right now, I don't want anyone else but me.

Lynda articulates a need of women across the ages, that of self-containment, a "room of one's own." In *Women and Madness*, psychotherapist and author Phyllis Chesler reveals in great detail how diffusing the self for the ease and pleasure of another can cause a complete disintegration of personality.[1] When a woman is able to rally from this extreme, it is usually with passion and fury—a passion that requires no other partner than herself.

Other times, sexual excess may lead to celibacy. Here is what Alena has to say:

> I was fairly repressed when I was young, living in a house that was immaculately clean and bound by strict rules of behavior. There was love, but there was also fear; I guess my mom was afraid of herself, and of us kids too, what we might do. I took the road less traveled (at least in my family) and dropped out of school. I met wild and wonderful people, and found I could make good money selling sexual favors…not prostitution exactly, but I'd give sexual massages, blow jobs, that kind of thing. I was choosy, though, and never a slave to anyone. For a while I felt free for the first time in my life. Then good friends turned bad, a few died of drug overdoses, and I turned to religion. I needed to purify myself, and I didn't have sex with anyone for three years.

As we enter our third decade of coping with STIs, stories like this become increasingly rare. Sexual addiction and overindulgence nonetheless remain pathways to celibacy for a number of women.

More commonly, women choose celibacy because they feel prostituted in conventional relationships. Often this comes from repressing the pain of unmet needs and feeling ignored or belittled. As the relationship deteriorates, sex becomes sporadic: a few encounters here and there, and then weeks with no contact. Interestingly, research has shown that sporadic sexual activity is more likely to cause menstrual irregularity and subfertility than is celibacy. Masturbation (even to orgasm) does not seem to compensate. Either regular sex, or none at all, tends to maintain normal hormonal levels and rhythms.[2]

Unless a couple has an agreement to the contrary, nothing disrupts sexual closeness like infidelity. Trust is so basic to a healthy relationship that if it is violated, intimacy may be impossible to regain without separation and time to heal. Again, a classic account, from Harriet:

> *My husband was unfaithful from day one, but it took me years to acknowledge this. Once I did, I went crazy with jealousy and fear. I started having anxiety attacks; I just couldn't control myself. I'd be at the bank or in some store, and suddenly I'd feel dizzy, breathless, light-headed—my heart would be racing and I'd have to sit down.*
>
> *I ended my marriage, but then, the same thing happened with the next guy. I finally realized that sex had become so fearsome and painful for me that I'd probably keep losing again and again, unless I broke the cycle on my own. So I quit looking for the right man, for perfect romance, and got down to being by myself. Some days I felt so alone that the panic nearly got me again, but eventually I could catch these feelings and get rid of them right away. I discovered things that nourished me and made me feel complete, instead of trying to fit other people's notions of what I should be.*

Pain and heartbreak aside, it is time for women to recognize that the sexes definitely differ in erotic temperament. According to research presented in *Brain Sex,* there is convincing evidence that men are by nature polygamous and tend to focus on sex for its own sake.[3] This does not preclude romance or even monogamous commitment, but a woman should know what she is dealing with if partnered with a male. Happiness comes not from seeking an idealized version of masculinity, but in accepting men as they are. Relationships involve conflict because male and female desires appear to be at odds, but they may also be viewed as complementary. Each has gender-based needs that are fairly consistent; John Gray has illuminated this quite well. For example, women need to feel cared for and loved in order to be able to trust their partners. Men need to feel trusted in order to care; a man without a woman's trust loses his momentum and vitality. Men will invariably fail to care for us as we would like, and we will likewise lose trust in them, but that doesn't change the basic needs of each. The more realistic we are about our differences, and the more we accept our own tendencies, the better we will be at weathering the ups and downs in relationships, the inevitable challenges and disappointments.

When a woman chooses sexual abstinence, she has an opportunity to own both her masculine and feminine aspects and bring them to terms with each other. For example, she can look at how much love and nourishment she gives herself, and, if minimal, the resulting lack of vulnerability and trust she is able to offer others. This will not change her basic needs in a relationship—no matter how well she has learned to care for herself, she will still be susceptible to being hurt by an uncaring partner. But she may be better equipped to deal with disappointments and estrangement when they occur, and go on caring for herself regardless.

A period of abstinence is usually the most constructive if it is deliberate, as negative side effects such as depression are less likely to occur. If depression does enter the picture, watch for signs that it is worsening—lack of motivation, flat moods, or disinterest in personal hygiene. Counseling can help, as can getting out socially.

One reason women do not find much cultural support for celibacy is that men find sex a prerequisite for emotional release, a precursor to love. Women, on the other hand, are more readily able to love themselves and others without sexual demonstration. When women choose celibacy, they threaten male needs and male control; we see this reflected in our language by terminology that is far from flattering, such as *old maid*, *spinster*, and *prude*.

Thus some women worry about remaining physically attractive without the benefits of sexual contact. But celibacy does not preclude pleasuring yourself, and masturbation offers numerous benefits, not the least of which is stress relief. It also stimulates pelvic circulation, which helps keep the pelvic organs in good health. Then again, there are innumerable ways to find physical and emotional release unrelated to sex. Some women just don't want sex, whatever the reason, and that's all there is to it.

What, if any, are the physical effects of long-term abstinence? Although some women report symptoms of pelvic tension like chronic backache, increased PMS, or menstrual difficulties, just as many report cessation of these problems, particularly when abstinent after ending a miserable relationship. Women occasionally report losing touch with the monthly cycle, becoming less aware of fertile and premenstrual signals. If fertility awareness was used as a contraceptive method, this is certainly understandable. Perhaps women who think they have lost touch are subconsciously revising emotional and spiritual aspects of cycling to suit their newfound autonomy.

Many women notice increased awareness of diet and health when on their own. Without the distraction of caring for another, they are better able to see the results of their own nutrition and lifestyle habits, and to experiment with what makes them feel best. Particularly if a woman has been living with someone and cooking and eating more to suit his or her wishes than her own, she may find this aspect of being alone most illuminating and beneficial.

Women often report that the less sex they have, the less they think about it. At times, the longing for contact is strong, but it may be more a desire for intimacy than for sex itself. Celibacy is really less about sex than it is about autonomy, learning to deal with one's own body, psyche, and soul.

Other reasons why a woman might choose to avoid sex temporarily have little to do with relationship. A friend recently shared plans for a yearlong trip around the world, along with her decision to forego sexual involvement until after she left—no dates, no serious flirting, just packing and settling affairs. Similar motivations might be found in plans to relocate, change careers, or focus on a creative project. When taken as a spiritual discipline, celibacy has long been reputed to enhance energy and concentration.

What if a woman elects to take this option in spite of the fact that she is in relationship? Although we hear much about varying degrees of desire between partners, the desire for periodic abstinence is at last out of the closet. Surveys on sexual frequency in committed relationships can be intimidating and discouraging of this, but remember, these surveys deal in averages only; they do not address the quality of sexual interactions, nor do they exclude the flurry of activity typical in the early stages of relationship when major challenges to intimacy have yet to be faced. I can think of no long-term study that truly reflects phases of closeness and separation in enduring relationships.

How does a couple get by when one wants sex and the other does not? Ideally, they discuss the matter, make some agreements, and set some limits. If this does not work, they need outside help. Relationships in distress are frequently challenged to redefine sex from an obligatory or perfunctory activity to one based on free will. Periodic abstinence may be crucial to sorting out individual needs and rhythms. So much more the case if either partner has been unfaithful, or emotionally or physically abusive. After all, what possible tenderness, joy, or security could come from sexual contact under such tenuous circumstances?

Sometimes the desire for abstinence becomes permanent, as in Joan's case:

> I'm sixty-nine now, and my husband died six years ago. A couple of years after his death, friends tried to set me up with men, and at first I was curious, interested. But each time it was so obviously wrong that all I felt was revulsion. I'd think to myself, "I have to get in bed with that?" I had such a wonderful marriage, and now I have my children and grandchildren. I've got used to being alone, and honestly, I like it.

At the other end of spectrum is the desire to wait for the right relationship. More women are choosing to remain virgins late into their teens or throughout their early twenties, which has much to do with living in the shadow of AIDS and other sexually transmitted infections. Others may have had a number of relationships and may continue to date, and yet choose to wait for the right partner to have sex.

For the first time in modern history, women have the freedom to choose from a spectrum of sexual options. Now that sex by coercion is defined as abuse, and sex by obligation is becoming passé, we are free to acknowledge ourselves as sexual beings, even if celibate. The prime dictum of sex therapy—"Don't worry about pleasing your partner, start by pleasing yourself"—may soon be realized by women on a mass scale. Women will find that their sexual energy is vital to their own well-being, instrumental to their creativity, health, and happiness, whether shared with another or not. Indeed, it will seem increasingly natural and normal that a woman (or man) might have times in life when sexual interaction is either inappropriate, undesirable, or low on the list of priorities, or that there will be times when we elect to channel our sexual energy into personal pursuits.

CHAPTER 11

○

Your Own Rhythms

How you make use of the material in this book depends on many things, not the least of which are any unresolved issues of abuse, grief, or loss. These so strongly affect your receptivity and sense of self that they will almost certainly overshadow the usual changes at different stages of life.

And yet, with daily observation, we may begin to notice the patterns and cycles in our lives, as well as ways in which we are consistently troubled or inhibited: our toughest challenges. The more creatively and constructively we are able to work on these, the richer and more multidimensional our experience at the next stage of life will be.

This closing chapter is written workbook style, with questions intended to shed light on your personal psychosexual patterns and how these extrapolate to rhythms of desire. Rather than allow blank space for writing within the book, I encourage you to use separate paper. The questions are provocative; I doubt you would want someone browsing through your bookshelves to come across your responses.

But do write your answers down! Committing yourself in writing is altogether different from musing, even if aloud. As you write, you may notice certain words that keep cropping up, or phrases from the treasure box of your past that have deep and vivid meaning for you. Or you may find empty expressions that you might wish to rethink or change.

Your journey through the labyrinth of sexuality is not only personal; it is also mythic. Don't be afraid to lend this dimension of value and significance to the intimate details of your life.

Sexual Awakening

◎

See if you can get in touch with your history here, tracing back your sexual attitudes, inhibitions, and expectations. Go back to the beginning: How did you learn about sex? Were you given a chance to question as fully as you desired? How did those you questioned respond to you? Do you remember the first time you masturbated? What was your first orgasm like? How was your first experience of sexual experimentation with another, and your first experience of penetration by another? How did you feel about each of these experiences?

How did you learn about menstruation? What was your menarche like—was it hidden from the rest of your family and friends, or acknowledged in some positive way?

You may wish to recast these events in a more positive framework. Even if you had no celebration at your menarche, it is never too late. What would you like this celebration to include? I know a woman who recently crafted and held a menarche rite for herself, at the age of forty-one!

If your first experience of sexual experimentation, masturbation, or penetration by another was guilt-ridden or demeaning, rewrite the script. Take who you are and what you know now, then draft a vision of how these events might have taken place in a way that would have been more to your liking. You may wish to share this with someone special—maybe your partner or a good friend—so that your revision is witnessed.

Discovering Your Cycle

◎

If you are just now learning about your monthly cycle, certain emotions will probably arise. Most women wonder why no one ever told them these facts about sex and their bodies before. Do you feel angry at having been kept in the dark this way? Or do you feel foolish or inept for never having noticed your own cyclic changes? Or perhaps you simply feel loss and sadness at having missed out on this aspect of yourself for some period of time. Typically, women are both disturbed and affirmed to find that romantic feelings attributed to a particular relationship were in large part biological promptings coming from their own bodies at certain times of the month.

You may wish to go back through the questions in the previous paragraph and examine your feelings more closely, exploring them a bit in writing. Try to evoke the curious, courageous you, unfettered by guilt or fear, confidently following your own lead.

Choose this, or another power image of yourself, and bring it to the task at hand: discovering and trusting your cycle. If you are troubled with PMS, irregular or painful menses, or infertility that has no apparent physical cause, ask your wise self for counsel. Do this in writing, meditation, or dreams.

If you feel completely out of touch, can't remember anything, or are upset by this exercise, refer to Chapter 9, particularly the list on page 190 of charcteristics common in abused women.

If your cycle is basically smooth and trouble-free, take a moment to consider why. Do you follow any particular menstrual routine or ritual? Cultural mores view menstrual blood on a spectrum from filthy to sacred. How do you feel about your blood? Do you enjoy and make the most of your fertile time? How so? How do you benefit most from paying attention to your cycle? And what do you have yet to learn and do to more fully honor your rhythms?

If you feel you are fairly complete with this area of investigation, single out any aspects that remain troublesome or unsettled for you. These are your carryover issues. As you move through the next stages, you will be able to view these issues in new contexts, which may help you better cope with them.

Pregnant for the First Time

◎

Having your first baby? Then you have much to contemplate and decide. You may have already discovered that pregnancy is a social event. You are probably being bombarded with questions, advice, or even physical contact (belly touching) from absolute strangers. This, you can't avoid. In fact, if you are able to stay open and objective, you may use these encounters to learn more about your beliefs and conditioning, particularly if you feel yourself being triggered by another's words or actions.

Let's look at your background more closely. What did your mother tell you about birth? How did you react? What about your grandmother or other female relatives? Try to recollect your feelings at these moments of revelation. If you were to summon each of these women now to stand before you, what sort of wisdom might each impart about how to cope with labor?

Control is a major issue in childbearing. How do you feel about losing control? About being and appearing vulnerable? How do you think you might behave if the pain really got to you? What kinds of things could your partner or care provider do to help you feel better? What could you do to help yourself? Do any of these relate to your sensual and sexual likes and dislikes?

Look at the last few questions, and see if there are any revelations you can share with your partner or care provider. For example, maybe you love to have your hair stroked, or your head held, or your feet rubbed, but nobody knows this except you. Pregnancy is the time to make these desires known, absolutely.

Fantasize about yourself in labor. Where are you? Is it dark, light, noisy, or quiet? Who is with you, and what are they doing? What are you doing? What position are you in, how are you breathing, and how do you feel?

Now imagine your labor suddenly getting much stronger. Wow—it really hurts! How do you react? Do you open up, or close down? Do you reach out for help, or go deep within? Relate these responses to your experience of sex. What do you do when it stops feeling good, either emotionally or physically? Women sometimes think they must continue with sex even though they feel themselves shutting down. Think about the times this has happened to you. What was it you really wanted? Crack the code on this matter, and you will discover the kind of support you are most likely to need in labor.

How do you handle being sexually frustrated? Do you ask for what you want, get angry, sulk, or withdraw? Take the opportunity while pregnant to begin asking for what you need, when you need it, in every possible area of your life, and especially in bed. This is core preparation for giving birth.

Finally, how do you respond when others try to tell you what's good for you? Do you clam up and keep the peace, become angry, or assert your position? With regard to extraneous advice during labor, or procedures you do not want, how do you think you might respond? What do you think would be most effective?

Pregnant Again?

◎

Whether carrying your second, third, or fourth baby, you will probably have issues remaining from your other birth experiences that merit attention. Did you feel in any way violated during your birth experience? Were things done to you or the baby without your permission or that you did not desire? Was your privacy invaded? Did you feel powerless, unsupported, ridiculed, or ridiculous in a way you can't let go of? Did your care provider break promises he or she made to you? Do you feel that he or she abandoned you during or after the birth?

If any of the above fit, you may want to write a letter to the appropriate party or parties. Whether you choose to send it or not, writing it will be therapeutic. I personally think it is critical to let your care provider know how you feel—critical for you, for them, and for all the women they serve.

How was your partner during the whole experience? Did he or she let you down or disappoint you in any way? Do you have feelings about what happened between you during labor that you have never shared? Did the birth affect your sex life or intimacy? Again, a letter is a good place to start; it can help you sort through your thoughts and feelings before you begin to discuss them.

If your partner's behavior during the birth links to some long-term problem that the two of you have been over many times, you may be ripe for counseling. Perhaps you see the need, but can you assert it to your partner? If not, you may be bound by feelings of unworthiness or a lack of self-esteem. Perhaps you have a history of abuse. You need support and an opportunity to express yourself, either one-on-one with a counselor or in group therapy.

Don't wait to begin this work—do it now. Read widely, and educate yourself on your birth options. Communicate your hopes and desires to your partner and care provider, and your next experience could be the birth of your dreams!

Newly Postpartum

◎

If you are newly or recently postpartum, you may be struggling with feelings of dependency. Often these arise during labor, although you may not have recognized them as such. Feelings of dependency are strongly linked to fears of abandonment.

Let us not confuse dependency with vulnerability. Vulnerability is normal in labor; it is actually a desired state, characterized by high levels of sensitivity, openness, and receptivity. In contrast, dependency is marked by feelings of not being able to rely on yourself, of needing others to define your reality.

Hospital policies and personnel often engender feelings of dependency in patients so they will be compliant. Highly invasive or unnecessary procedures exacerbate these feelings. If a woman feels that she has lost her power in labor, she will likely feel abandoned by those who stood by and let it happen. Or she may feel that it was all her fault.

Here are some questions to help you sort out this out. Did you make your best attempt to educate yourself during pregnancy, and to set up your birth situation in advance? Did you inform those on your birth team—your partner, care provider, and other intimates—of your plans and wishes? If so, work through your disappointment as suggested in the previous section, or just let it be—it is certainly not your fault.

Or perhaps you found it hard to focus on your own needs while pregnant. Did you feel less and less communicative as pregnancy progressed? If things were done during labor that you did not want, did you feel like it was your fault? Do you often feel that everyone has power but you? Do you find yourself becoming deeply upset or anxious if people pull away from or reject you? Affirmative answers to these questions link strongly to a history of abuse. Get help for this.

Regarding the postpartum period, there is yet another category of abuse to consider: that which is perpetrated by society. In Chapter 5, we looked at the routine abandonment of new mothers in the United States. Even women who have led relatively stable lives may find themselves exhibiting symptoms of anxiety and depression at this juncture. Generally, the solution is as much a matter of practical assistance with recovery and household responsibilities as of emotional support.

But some women are barely able to tolerate the vulnerability of motherhood. Before the birth, did you resolve that your baby would disrupt your life as little as possible? Did you choose to have medication early in labor? When you first held your baby, did you have any feelings of ambivalence? Were (or are) you anxious to get back to work at once? Fear of motherhood is often linked to limited love and affection in childhood. What was your mother's approach to child rearing? Did she set good boundaries, or was she self-sacrificing? What were her views of menstruation, childbearing, and sexuality? As you care for your baby, do you often feel upset or at the breaking point? If so, frustration can build to dangerous levels and may lead to violence. Get help. Make an anonymous call to a women's hotline or counseling referral service as soon as possible.

We have already discussed postpartum sexual frustrations. Are you compounding these with negative feelings about your body? Do you find your copious secretions (milk, lochia, sweat) offensive? Do you feel ashamed that you look a bit softer and plumper than usual? Or do you take pride in your body for all it has accomplished: birth, breast-feeding, day-by-day recovery, and care of your newborn?

Has your weight been an issue for most of your adult life? If so, you will probably be unhappy postpartum. Do you have a history of eating disorders? Nothing is worse for you and your baby than dieting while breast-feeding; in fact, you need more calories than you did while pregnant. Exercise is the answer, even though it takes a while to find the time and energy for a workout.

A few other considerations: Do you feel any conflict between being a mother and being sexual? Where do you think this comes from? What were your mother's beliefs in this regard? What are your partner's attitudes on the subject? At first, it feels awkward to swing so dramatically from erotic to maternal feelings, but as the baby grows and privacy returns, these feelings settle into their respective places.

The primary question postpartum is this: Can you give yourself permission to change and grow? Do you trust your body to tell you what to eat and drink, and when to rest? Do you believe that your body will fully recover in good time? Or do you feel that your body has betrayed you? Have others told you that your body is not up to par, not good enough? Think of every individual who has told you this throughout your lifetime, and explore your response to each. Can you let go of your anger and love yourself?

Keep a journal of your daily accomplishments at this stage. Pay special attention to the times you feel physically well and wonderful, and write about them, too.

Juggling Career, Family, and Intimacy
◎

The work to be done in the area of juggling a career, a family, and intimacy can probably be summed up in a single question: What are your priorities? You may be able to learn more about our own values if you examine the priorities of your parents. Are you emulating or reacting to them, or are you truly self-determined?

How was it in your household? Was your mother enmeshed in trying to do too much? What messages did you get from your parents regarding their respective responsibility for housework? What about responsibility for the children? Who took responsibility for emotional issues? Was there individual responsibility for health and well-being, or did Mom handle it all?

What was your mother's attitude regarding her own needs? Did she take private time? What were the things she loved to do, just for herself? Did she set boundaries that you and other family members were aware of and respected?

Generally, women tend to make care of the children their top priority, and that is as it should be. But did your mother have any help? What kind, and how often? Do you think it was enough?

This brings us to the subjects of stress and anger. How did your mother handle these emotions? How do you handle them? How does your approach to stress and anger affect you and your loved ones?

What was your parents' attitude about their intimate relationship? Did they show their feelings for each other? Did they make time for their love, apart from you? How open were your parents about sexual matters? What was the basic attitude or feeling about sex in your household? Were your personal boundaries and need for privacy respected by your family?

Take a look at your current weekly commitments. You may benefit from writing down all that you do, and then calculating the amount of time spent in areas of career, housework, family time, personal time, and private time with your partner. Play with this on paper: Look at any obvious imbalance, and reallocate your time to suit your needs right now. Many of us believe ourselves to be trapped by necessity in unsatisfying time commitments, when in fact these are simply a matter of habit. Women at this stage of life must recognize that there will never be enough time to do and have it all. Your priorities can and should change from day to day, week to week, month to month, year to year. Consider developing a one-year plan, five-year plan, and ten-year plan as a means to be more in touch with your purpose in life.

If this seems extremely difficult for you, look back at the questions in this chapter that concern your self-esteem. Do you see patterns of putting yourself down or setting your own needs aside? Perhaps if you can determine when and to whom you give up your power, you will be able to figure out why.

Passing Through Menopause

◎

As mentioned in Chapter 7, your responses as you pass through menopause are likely to reflect those of female relatives, particularly your mother. What did she experience at menopause? Is there anything about her experience that you personally remember? Since most women tend to hide their symptoms, you may want to ask her about any erratic behavior you recall and see what the two of you can piece together.

Moving to yet another area: How do you feel about the passing of your youth? Do you see youth as a state of mind, one that can be maintained indefinitely? If so, what are you doing to keep yourself young and vital? How well are you keeping up with your own interests? How about your spiritual life?

How are you caring for your body at this point? Take inventory of all that you do to stay fit and attractive. Truthfully, are any of these practices a waste of time and money? What does seem to work for you, and how can you place greater emphasis on it?

Have you talked to your partner about your fears and anxieties at this stage of life? Has she or he been supportive? As the hormonal surges of menopause move you ever closer to your deepest concerns and longings, do you find that you can share these with your partner? And how do you use your visions? Are you incorporating them into your life, or merely coping?

Think about where you want to go after "the change." Can you use your menopausal energy as a springboard to expand your life? Who are your closest allies in this process? How can you make the most of the support they offer?

Growing Older and Wiser

◎

How do you feel about growing older? What do you still look forward to experiencing or accomplishing? What about your partner? Have you discussed your rounding-out goals and dreams with one another?

What lessons do you have yet to learn in life? Are there challenging situations that keep repeating themselves? What will it take for you to move through them? Can you deliberately set the stage for this, and to what degree are you willing to do so? Who are your best allies for confronting these challenges?

With regard to sex: How is your communication with your partner? Are you happy with yourself sexually: more or less so than before? In terms of sexual self-expression, are there things you would still like to try? How do you think your partner would react?

Look closely at yourself now, and look back to where you have been. Are there ways you still don't feel comfortable with your body? Are there parts of your body you never learned to love? Are there sexual wounds or criticisms you have never healed? See whether or not you need to be witnessed, or if you can find a way to embrace yourself fully on your own. In terms of longevity, a healthy body is an integrated body.

How are your relationships with your grown children? Are you comfortable sharing ideas with them, or do you feel misplaced? Identify your Crone aspect: wise, objective, and irrevocably frank. When the Crone speaks, she does so from a point of clarity and certitude. Feel the difference between whining or cajoling and speaking the truth, without expectations.

Do you have many outlets for your accumulated wisdom? Can you find any more? Your vitality is strongly linked to your self-expression.

Have you considered taking the role of family historian? If you have not done so already, you might begin assembling and organizing papers and photographs into albums, adding your own narrative if you like. Each of your children can have a personal album, and you may also want to create a composite that includes the family tree. All of these will be treasured by your offspring, and creating them will give you some closure in certain areas of your life.

In Summary

◎

Now that you have had the opportunity to reflect on each phase of life you've already experienced and have read about others yet to come, perhaps you have discovered some underlying theme in your sexual story, woven from your family history, ways that culture has affected you, and all you have done on your path of self-discovery. Remember the definition of sexuality given earlier: For a woman, sexuality is all that it means to be female. This is the key to both pleasure and intimacy—bringing all of yourself to your sexual encounters.

Our journey as women through this particular period of history is tremendously rich and complex. Keeping an overview of the cycles and stages in life can help us keep our wits about us, retain a sense of humor, and become wise. And, as men become more concerned with finding balance in their own lives, it has never been more important, or in many ways easier, to articulate all that it means to be a woman.

But we have a long way to go. Far too many women live in poverty, abusive situations, or other conditions of hardship for us to become complacent. We have so much to do, so much to speak and write about, and so much to share across the generations. May our sexual vitality infuse these tasks with passion, commitment, and love. And may we find courage at every crossroads.

Women's Worksheet on Abuse and Trauma

To get the most from this worksheet, please answer these questions as honestly as possible (using separate paper or a photocopy). Your responses are meant to stimulate self-reflection and increased awareness of factors that may influence your self-esteem and intimate relationships. If you are disturbed by any of your findings, contact a counselor for assistance.

Did you suffer physical or emotional neglect as a child? What have you done to address this?

_____

_____

_____

_____

How does this affect you now?

_____

_____

_____

_____

Have you suffered physical or emotional neglect as an adult? What have you done to address this?

_____

_____

_____

_____

What is your situation now?

_____

_____

_____

_____

Have you ever been in an abusive relationship (physically and/or emotionally intimidated, beaten, or injured)? What have you done to address this?

_____

_____

_____

_____

What is your situation now?

_____

_____

_____

_____

Have you ever been molested or had nonconsensual sex with a partner, relative, or acquaintance? What have you done to address this?

_____

_____

_____

_____

What is your situation now?

_____

_____

_____

_____

Have you ever been promiscuous or sexually careless on a regular basis? What have you done to address this?

_____

_____

_____

_____

What is your situation now?

_____

_____

_____

_____

Have you ever been raped? What have you done to address this?

_____

_____

_____

_____

How does this affect you now?

_____

_____

_____

_____

Have ever been subject to gynecological or obstetrical abuse? What have you done to address this?

_____

_____

_____

_____

How does this affect you now?

_____

_____

_____

_____

Have you ever had anorexia, bulimia, or eating problems? What have you done to address this?

_____

_____

_____

_____

What is your situation now?

_____

_____

_____

_____

Do you think, or has anyone ever told you, that you have used alcohol or recreational drugs excessively? What have you done to address this?

_____

_____

_____

_____

Does this continue to be an issue?

_____

_____

_____

_____

The following is a list of stressors that can impact your physical and emotional health as well as your sexuality: They can cause trauma that may remain deeply rooted. On a scale of 1 to 10 (with 10 being the greatest intensity), how high was your stress level in response to these occurrences?

_____ serious money problems (date/year) _____

_____ was a caregiver to someone ill or impaired (date/year)_____

_____ sudden death of a loved one (date/year)_____

_____ parents separated/divorced (date/year)_____

_____ separated/divorced (date/year)_____

_____ witnessed domestic violence (date/year)_____

_____ family member jailed (date/year)_____

_____ jailed (date/year)_____

_____ lived in war zone (date/year)_____

_____ sexually harassed (date/year)_____

_____ saw robbery or attack (date/year)_____

_____ robbed/attacked (date/year)_____

_____ painful medical procedure (date/year)_____

_____ saw accident (date/year)_____

_____ had accident (date/year)_____

_____ was in serious disaster (date/year/location)_____

_____ had a hard time with elective abortion or miscarriage
(date/year)_____

If you have experienced any other significant stressors, rate and date
them:

_____

_____

_____

(Regarding the stress index, acknowledgements to Mickey Sperlich
for her excellent article, "Survivor Moms: Multiple Trauma Expo-
sures and the Development of Posttraumatic Stress Disorder," *Midwifery Today* 90 (Summer 2009): 32–34.)

Notes

Author's Note

1. Helen Fisher, *The First Sex* (New York: Ballantine Books, 2001), 7.
2. Ibid, xvi.

Chapter 1

1. Nancy Friday, *Women on Top* (New York: Pocket Books, 1993), 34.
2. Natalie Angier, *Woman: An Intimate Geography* (New York: Anchor Books, 1999), 70.
3. Sheila Kitzinger, *Woman's Experience of Sex* (New York: Penguin Books, 1985), 39.
4. William H. Masters, and Virginia E. Johnson, *Human Sexual Response* (Boston, MA: Little, Brown, 1966).
4. Hallie Iglehart, *Woman Spirit* (San Francisco: Harper & Row, 1983), 9–10.
5. Barbara Walker, *The Crone* (San Francisco: Harper & Row, 1985), 46.
6. Susan Griffin, *Pornography and Silence* (New York: Harper & Row, 1982).
7. *Webster's New Collegiate Dictionary*, (1969), s.v. "sexuality."
8. Anne Moir and David Jessel, *Brain Sex* (New York: Carol Publishing Group, 1991), 18.
9. Camille Paglia, quoted in "Hurricane Camille Wreaks Havoc," *San Francisco Chronicle,* September, 1992.
10. Moir and Jessel, *Brain Sex*, 42–43.
11. Christiane Northrup, *Women's Bodies, Women's Wisdom,* rev. ed. (New York: Bantam, 2010), 34.
12. Laura S. Allen et al., "Sexual Dimorphism of the Anterior Commissure and the Massa Intermedia of the Human Brain," *Journal of Comparative Neurology* 312 (1991): 97–104; Laura S. Allen et al., "Sex Differences in the Corpus Callosum of the Living Human Being," *Journal of Neuroscience* 11, no. 4 (1991): 933–42, http://www.jneurosci.org/content/11/4/933 (accessed 15 November 2012).
13. John Gray, *Men, Women and Relationships* (New York: Fine Communications, 2001), 80.

Chapter 2

1. Carol Gilligan, *In a Different Voice: Psychological Theory of Women's Development* (Cambridge, MA: Harvard University Press, 1993), xxii–xxiii.

2. Joan Borysenko, *Reflections on a Woman's Book of Life* (Carlsbad, CA: Hay House Audio Books, 1997), audiotape.
3. Gilligan, *In a Different Voice*, 51.
4. Elizabeth Davis and Carol Leonard, *The Women's Wheel of Life* (New Hampshire: Bad Beaver Publishing, 2012), 112.
5. Theresa L. Crenshaw, *The Alchemy of Love and Lust* (New York: Pocket Books, 1997), 31.
6. Natalie Angier, *Woman: An Intimate Geography* (New York: Anchor Books, 1999), 15.
7. Robin Baker, *Sperm Wars: Infidelity, Sexual Conflict, and Other Bedroom Battles* (New York: Basic Books, 2006), 197.
8. Angier, *Woman: An Intimate Geography,* 66.
9. Ibid, 53.
10. David Cohen, *The Circle of Life* (New York: HarperCollins, 1993), 64.
11. Ibid, 62.

Chapter 3

1. Ivana Hromatko, "The Influence of Estrogen on Spatial Ability, Perceptual Speed and Fine Motor Abilities," *Contemporary Psychology* 4 (December 2001).
2. Antonella Gasbarri et al., "Estrogen and Cognitive Functions," *Expert Review of Endocrinology and Metabolism* 5, no. 5 (2009): 507–520.
3. Winnifred B. Cutler, *Love Cycles* (New York: Villard Books, 1991), 177.
4. Christiane Northrup, *Women's Bodies, Women's Wisdom,* rev. ed. (New York: Bantam Books, 2010), 105.
5. Fisher, *The First Sex,* 129.
6. Joan Borysenko, *Reflections on a Woman's Book of Life* (Carlsbad, CA: Hay House Audio Books, 1997), audiotape.
7. Lea Barton, "How to Remove Xenoestrogens,"eHow.com, 2012, http://www.ehow.com/how_4449304_remove-xenoestrogens.html (accessed 15 October 2012).
8. Theresa L. Crenshaw, *The Alchemy of Love and Lust* (New York: Pocket Books, 1997), 6.
9. Barbara G. Walker, *The Woman's Encyclopedia of Myths and Secrets* (San Francisco: Harper & Row, 1995), 643.
10. Judy Grahn, *Blood, Bread, and Roses* (Boston, MA: Beacon Press, 1994), 52.
11. Dena Taylor, *Red Flower: Rethinking Menstruation* (Caldwell, NJ: Blackburn Press, 2003).
12. Penelope Shuttle and Peter Redgrove, *The Wise Wound* (London: Marion Boyars Publishers, 2005), 96.
13. Taylor, *Red Flower.*

14. Crenshaw, *The Alchemy of Love and Lust,* 101.
15. Mary Jane Sherfey, *The Nature and Evolution of Female Sexuality* (New York: Random House, 1973), 52.
16. Walker, *The Woman's Encyclopedia of Myths and Secrets,* 640–41.
17. Northrup, *Women's Bodies, Women's Wisdom,* 123–26.
18. Luisa Francia, *Dragontime* (New York: Ash Tree Publishing, 1991).
19. FDA STUDY 313-NA, www.accessdata.fda.gov/drugsatfda_docs/label /2008/021864s002lbl.pdf (accessed 4 February 2013).
20. Tarek Bardawil and Alberto Manetta, "Vaginal Cancer," http://emedicine. medscape.com/article/269188-overview (accessed May 5, 2012).
21. Rosemarie Krug et. al., "Selective Influence of Menstrual Cycle on Perception of Stimuli with Reproductive Significance," *Psychosomatic Medicine* 56 (1994): 410–17.
22. C. Wedekind et al., "MHC-Dependent Mate Preferences in Humans," in *Proceedings of the Royal Society of London* 22, no. 1359 (1995): 245–49, http://www.ncbi.nlm.nih.gov/pubmed/7630893 (accessed 15 November 2012).
23. S. Sumiala et al., "Salivary Progesterone Concentration After Tubal Sterilization," *Obstetrics and Gynecology* 88 (1996): 792–96.

Chapter 4

1. Niles Newton and Charlotte Modahl, "New Frontiers of Oxytocin Research," in *Free Woman: Women's Health in the 1990s,* eds. E. V. Van Hall and W. Everaerd (Canforth, England: Parthenon Publishing Group, 1989).
2. Ina May Gaskin, *Spiritual Midwifery,* 4th ed. (Summertown, TN: Book Publishing Co., 2002), 60.
3. Niles Newton, Donald Foshee, and Michael Newton, "Experimental Inhibition of Labor Through Environmental Disturbance," *Obstetrics and Gynecology* 27, no. 3 (1966): 371–77, http://www.ncbi.nlm.nih.gov /pubmed/5909557 (accessed 15 November 2012).
4. Grantly Dick-Read, *Childbirth Without Fear* (New York: Harper & Row, 1959), 158–60.
5. United Nations Statistics Division http://unstats.un.org (search neonatal mortality).
6. World Health Organization, http://apps.who.int/gho/data/?vid=2500 (accessed 4 February 2013).
7. Kenneth Johnson and Betty-Anne Daviss, "Outcomes of Planned Hospital Births with Certified Midwives: A Large Prospective Study in North America," *British Medical Journal* 330, no. 7505 (2005): 1416, http://www.ncbi .nlm.nih.gov/pmc/articles/PMC558373 (accessed 15 November 2012).
8. Patricia A. Janssen et al., "Outcomes of Planned Home Birth with Registered Midwife versus Planned Hospital Birth with Midwife or Physician,"

Canadian Medical Association Journal 181, no. 6–7 (August 2009): 377–83, http://www.ncbi.nlm.nih.gov/pmc/articles/PMC2742137 (accessed 15 November 2012).

9. Eileen K. Hutton, Angela H. Reitsma, and Karyn Kaufman, "Outcomes Associated with Planned Home and Planned Hospital Births in Low-Risk Women Attended by Midwives in Ontario, Canada, 2003–2006: A Retrospective Cohort Study," *Birth* 36, no. 3 (September 2009): 180–89.

10. Sheila Kitzinger, *Woman's Experience of Sex* (New York: Penguin Books, 1985), 217–18.

11. Michel Odent, *Water and Sexuality* (London: Penguin Books, 1990), 8.

12. Roberto Caldeyro-Barcia, "The Influence of Maternal Bearing-down Efforts During Second Stage on Fetal Well-being," *Birth and the Family Journal* 6, no. 1 (spring 1979).

13. E. B. Keverne et al., "Vaginal Stimulation: An Important Determinant of Maternal Bonding in Sheep," *Science* 219, no. 4580 (1983): 81–83, http://www.ncbi.nlm.nih.gov/pubmed/6849123 (accessed 15 November 2012).

14. D. Krehbiel et al., "Peridural Anesthesia Disturbs Maternal Behavior in Primiparous and Multiparous Parturient Ewes," *Physiology and Behavior* 40, no. 4 (1982): 463–72.

Chapter 5

1. Niles Newton and Charlotte Modahl, "Mood State Differences Between Breast and Bottle-Feeding Mothers," in *Newton on Breastfeeding* (Seattle, WA: Birth and Life Bookstore, 1990).

2. Evelyn B. Thoman, A. Wetzel, and S. Levine, "Lactation Prevents Disruption of Temperature Regulation and Suppresses Adrenocortical Activity in Rats," *Communicative Behavior in Biology* 2, part A (1968).

3. Niles Newton, "The Role of the Oxytocin Reflexes in Three Interpersonal Reproductive Acts: Coitus, Birth and Breastfeeding," in *Newton on Breastfeeding* (Seattle, WA: Birth and Life Bookstore, 1990).

4. Gloria Steinem, *Revolution from Within* (Boston: Little, Brown, 1993), 4–5.

5. William H. Masters and Virginia E. Johnson, *Human Sexual Response* (New York: Ishi Press, 2010), 168.

6. Kerstin Uvnäs-Moberg, "The Role of Efferent and Afferent Vagal Nerve Activity During Reproduction: Integrating Function of Oxytocin on Metabolism and Behavior," *Psychoneuroendocrinology* 19 (1994): 687–95.

Chapter 6

1. Camille Paglia, quoted in "Hurricane Camille Wreaks Havoc," *San Francisco Chronicle*, September, 1992.

2. Elizabeth Davis and Carol Leonard, *The Women's Wheel of Life* (Hopkinton, NH: Bad Beaver Publishing, 2012), 172.

3. John Gray, *Men, Women and Relationships* (New York: Fine Communications, 2001), 226.
4. M. F. Belenky et al., *Women's Ways of Knowing* (New York: Basic Books, 1997), 118, 144.
5. Marilyn Ruman, "Sex and Anger," *New Woman*, April 1991.
6. Gray, *Men, Women and Relationships*, 134.
7. Davis and Leonard, *The Women's Wheel of Life*, 136–37.
8. T. Berry Brazelton, *Infants and Mothers* (New York: Delacorte Press, 1983), 46.
9. Pepper Schwartz, *Peer Marriage: How Love Between Equals Really Works* (New York: The Free Press, 1995), 2, 3.
10. Andrew Ward, *Out Here* (New York: Penguin Books, 1991).
11. June Reinisch, "The Kinsey Report" (syndicated), *San Francisco Chronicle*, 1990.

Chapter 7

1. Robert A. Wilson, *Feminine Forever* (New York: Pocket Books, 1971), 19.
2. David Reuben, *Everything You Always Wanted to Know About Sex but Were Afraid to Ask* (New York: Bantam Books, 1971).
3. Sheila Kitzinger, *Woman's Experience of Sex* (New York: Penguin Books, 1985), 233.
4. Susan Lark, *The Menopause Self-Help Book* (Berkeley, CA: Celestial Arts, 2004), 36.
5. Joan Borysenko, *Reflections on a Woman's Book of Life* (Carlsbad, CA: Hay House Audio Books, 1997), audiotape.
6. As cited in Borysenko's *Reflections on a Woman's Book of Life*.
7. Writing Group for the Women's Health Initiative Investigators, "Risks and Benefits of Estrogen Plus Progestin in Healthy Postmenopausal Women: Principal Results from the Women's Health Initiative Randomized Controlled Trial," *Journal of the American Medical Association* 288, no. 3 (July 2002): 321–333, http://jama.jamanetwork.com/article.aspx?articleid=195120 (accessed 15 November 2012).
8. F. Grodstein et al., "Postmenopausal Hormone Therapy and Mortality," *New England Journal of Medicine* 336, no. 25 (1997): 1769–76, http://www.nejm.org/doi/full/10.1056/NEJM199706193362501 (accessed 15 November 2012).
9. Writing Group for the Women's Health Initiative Investigators, "Risks and Benefits of Estrogen Plus Progestin in Healthy Postmenopausal Women."
10. J. Jeppesen et al., "Effects of Low-Fat, High-Carbohydrate Diets on Risk Factors for Ischemic Heart Disease in Postmenopausal Women," *American Journal of Clinical Nutrition* 65, no. 4 (1997): 1027–33, http://ajcn.nutrition.org/content/65/4/1027.long (accessed 15 November 2012).

11. Barbara Sherwin, "The Use of Androgens in the Postmenopause — Evidence from Clinical Studies," *Maturitas* 27 (1996).

12. Rollin McCraty, "How Coherence Enhances Cognitive Function" webinar, www.heartmath.org (2010).

13. Elizabeth Davis and Carol Leonard, *The Women's Wheel of Life* (Hopkinton, NH: Bad Beaver Publishing, 2012), 173–74.

14. Susun Weed, *New Menopausal Years: The Wise Woman Way* (Portland, OR: Ash Tree Publishing, 2002).

15. Barbara Raskin, *Hot Flashes* (New York: St. Martin's Press, 1988).

16. Winnifred Culter, *Love Cycles* (New York: Villard Books, 1991), 42.

17. "Why Organic Food Matters," *The Journal of Sustainable Agriculture* 1, no. 1 (1985).

18. http://www.surgery.com/procedure/hysterectomy/demographics (2009) (accessed 4 February 2013).

19. Christiane Northrup, *Women's Bodies, Women's Wisdom,* rev. ed. (New York: Bantam Books, 2010), 527.

20. Dena Taylor, *Red Flower: Rethinking Menstruation* (Caldwell, NJ: Blackburn Press, 2003).

21. Barbara Walker, *The Crone* (San Francisco: Harper & Row, 1985), 51.

22. Zsuzsanna Budapest, *Holy Book of Women's Mysteries* (San Francisco, CA: Red Wheel/Weiser, 2007), 96–97.

Chapter 8

1. Barbara Walker, *The Crone* (San Francisco, CA: Harper & Row, 1985), 12–14.

2. Walker, *The Crone,* 126, 137.

3. Sheila Kitzinger, *Woman's Experience of Sex* (New York: Penguin Books, 1985), 238, 239.

4. Walker, *The Crone,* 31.

5. Natalie Angier, "Theorists See Evolutionary Advantages in Menopause," *New York Times* (September 1997).

6. Kristin Hawkes, J. F. O'Connell, and N. G. Burton, "The Grandmother Hypothesis and Human Evolution," in *Adaptation and Evolutionary Biology,* ed. L. Cronk et al. (New York: Aldine de Gruyter, forthcoming); Kristin Hawkes, J. F. O'Connell, and N. G. Burton, "Hadza Women's Time Allocation, Offspring Provisioning, and the Evolution of Long Postmenopausal Lifespans," *Current Anthropology* 38 (1997): 551–57.

7. Luisa Francia, *Dragontime* (New York: Ash Tree Publishing, 1991).

8. Rhonda L. Winn and Niles Newton, "Sexuality in Aging: A Study of 106 Cultures," *Archives of Sexual Behavior* 11, no. 4 (1982): 286–98.

9. Jerry Gerber et al., *Life Trends* (New York: Avon Books, 1991).

10. Ibid.

11. Ibid.
12. Sheila Kitzinger, *Woman's Experience of Sex* (New York: Penguin Books, 1985), 238.

Chapter 9

1. Her Majesty's Inspectorate of Constabulary, "Without Consent: A Report on the Joint Review of the Investigation and Prosecution of Rape Offences," (January 2007), http://www.hmic.gov.uk/media/without-consent-2006 1231.pdf (accessed 31 January 2013).
2. RAINN, "How Often Does Sexual Assault Occur?" http://www.rainn.org /get-information/statistics/frequency-of-sexual-assault (accessed 4 February 2013); "Rape Statistics—South Africa & Worldwide 2011," http:// www.rape.co.za/index.php?option=com_content&task=view&id=875 (accessed 4 February 2013).
3. Laura Davis and Ellen Bass, *The Courage to Heal* (New York: Vermillion, 1991).
4. Sheila Kitzinger, *Women's Experience of Sex* (New York: Penguin Books, 1985), 259.
5. Christiane Northrup, *Women's Bodies, Women's Wisdom,* rev. ed. (New York: Bantam Books, 2010), 93.
6. Mickey Sperlich and Julia Seng, *Survivor Moms* (Eugene, OR: Motherbaby Press, 2008), 197.
7. Beverly Engel, *The Emotionally Abused Woman* (New York, Random House, 1992), 22–27.
8. Avodah K. Offit, *The Sexual Self* (New York: J. B. Lippincott, 1977).
9. Engel, *The Emotionally Abused Woman,* 37.
10. Offit, *The Sexual Self.*
11. Robin Baker, *Sperm Wars: Infidelity, Sexual Conflict, and Other Bedroom Battles* (New York: Basic Books, 2006), xii–xiii.
12. Helen Fisher, *The First Sex: The Natural Talents of Women and How They Are Changing the World* (New York: Ballantine Books, 1999), 204.
13. Barbara Walker, *The Women's Encyclopedia of Myths and Secrets* (New York: HarperCollins, 1995), 653.

Chapter 10

1. Phyllis Chesler, *Women and Madness* (Hampshire, UK: Palgrave Macmillan, 2005).
2. Winnifred Cutler, *Love Cycles* (New York: Villard Books, 1991), 249.
3. A. Moir and D. Jessel, *Brain Sex* (New York: Carol Publishing, 1991), 105.

Index